Vaccination: A Tool for the Control of Avian Influenza

A joint OIE/FAO/IZSVe Conference supported by the European Commission

FAO FIAT PANIS

OIE World Organisation for Animal Health

IZSVe Istituto Zooprofilattico Sperimentale delle Venezie

••••••••••••••••••

Developments in Biologicals

Vol. 130

This series "Developments in Biologicals" begins vith vol.102 and is the continuation of IABS symposia series "Progress in Immunobiological Standardization", Vol 1-5, "Immunobiological Standardization", Vols 1-22 and "Developments in Biological Standardization", Vols 23-101.

Organized and published by the International Association for Biologicals (IABS)

KARGER

Basel . Freiburg . Paris . London . New York
Bangalore . Bangkok . Singapore . Tokyo . Sydney

Vaccination: A Tool for the Control of Avian Influenza

Verona, Italy
20-22 March, 2007

Volume editors *Betty Dodet*
Dodet Bioscience
Lyon, France

In collaboration with the Scientific and Technical Department of the OIE, Paris, France

Technical editor *Elisabeth Heseltine*

Proceedings of a joint OIE/FAO/IZSVe conference co-organised with the European Commission

6 figures and 24 tables, 2007

KARGER

Basel . Freiburg . Paris . London . New York
Bangalore . Bangkok . Singapore . Tokyo . Sydney

•••••••••••••••••

Developments in Biologicals

Library of Congress Cataloging-in-Publication Data

Joint OIE/FAO/IZSVe Conference "Vaccination: a Tool for the Control of Avian Influenza" (2007 : Verona, Italy)
Vaccination : a tool for the control of avian influenza : Verona, Italy, 20-22 March, 2007 : proceedings of a joint OIE/FAO/IZSVe conference co-organised with the European Commission / volume editors, Betty Dodet, in collaboration with the Scientific and Technical Department of the OIE, Paris, France ; technical editor, Elisabeth Heseltine.
p. ; cm. -- (Developments in biologicals ; v. 130)
Includes bibliographical references.
ISBN 978-3-8055-8484-5 (soft cover : alk. paper)
1. Avian influenza--Prevention--Congresses. 2. Poultry--Vaccination--Congresses. I. Dodet, Betty. II. International Office of Epizootics. Scientific and Technical Dept. III. Title. IV. Series.
[DNLM: 1. Influenza in Birds--prevention & control--Congresses. 2. Disease Outbreaks--prevention & control--Congresses. 3. Disease Outbreaks--veterinary--Congresses. 4. Influenza Vaccines--Congresses. 5. Vaccination--veterinary--Congresses. W1 DE997VKF v.130 2007 / SF 995.6.I6 J74v 2007]
SF995.6.I6J65 2007
636.5'0896203--dc22

2007050982

Bibliographic Indices. This publication is listed in bibliographic services, including Current Contents® and Index Medicus.

Drug dosage. The authors and the publisher have exerted every effort to ensure that drug selection and dosage set forth in this text are in accord with current recommendations and practice at the time of publication. However, in view of ongoing research, changes in government regulations, and the constant flow of information relating to drug therapy and drug reactions, the reader is urged to check the package insert for each drug for any change in indications and dosage and for added warnings and precautions. This is particularly important when the recommended agent is a new and/or infrequently employed drug.

Worldwide distribution by S. Karger AG, Basel (Switzerland).
Printed in France by IML, Saint-Matin-en-haut (France).
ISBN 978-3-8055-8484-5

The scientific integrity of the articles contained in this volume is the sole responsibility of the authors.

Steering Committee

G. Brückner (chairperson) (OIE)
J.L. Angot (OIE)
J. Domenech (FAO)
W. Schoustra (FAO)
S. Marangon (IZSVe)
A. Laddomada (EC)

Scientific Committee

C. Bruschke (chairperson) (OIE)
A. McLeod (FAO)
J. Lubroth (Co-chair) (FAO)
I. Capua (IZSVe)
M. Pittman (EC)
P. Jones (IFAH)
K. Stärk (Switzerland)
D. Swayne (USA)
Bui Quang Anh (Vietnam)
P. Daniels (Australia)
B. Seck (Mali)
D. Alexander (UK)

Acknowledgements

The joint OIE/FAO/IZSVe Conference "**Vaccination: A Tool for the control of Avian Influenza**" is grateful to the following organisations for their financial support:

National and International Organisations
European Commission
Italian Ministry of Health
The Province of Verona
The Veneto Region

Private Companies
INTERVET International B.V.
Merial Avian Global Enterprise
AIA Agricola Italiana Alimentare Spa
Con. Av. Consorzio Zoo-Avicunicolo
Boehringer Ingelheim Vetmedica
Laboratorio AVIMEX S.A de C.V.

Organisation of the Scientific Programme

Opening Session

Session I	Setting the Scene
Session II	Review of Experiences
Session III	Socioeconomic Effects of Vaccination
Session IV	Application of Vaccination
Session V	Vaccines and Research
Session VI	Regulatory and Trade Aspects
Session VII	Vaccination: an Integrated Approach
Session VIII	Conclusions and Recommendations

Contents

Dodet B and the Scientific & Technical Department of the OIE (eds): Vaccination: A Tool for the Control of Avian Influenza. Dev Biol (Basel). Basel, Karger, 2007, vol 130, pp XI-XII.

Preface

B. Vallat[1], *J. Domenech*[2], *S. Marangon*[3]

1 Director-General, World Organisation for Animal Health, Paris, France

2 Chief Veterinary Officer, Food and Agriculture Organization of the United Nations, Rome, Italy

3 Scientific Director, Istituto Zooprofilattico Sperimentale delle Venezie, Legnaro (Padova), Italy

During the past 3 years, the international community has faced the crisis of highly pathogenic avian influenza and its scientific, economic, political, social and ethical implications. The World Organisation for Animal Health (OIE) and the Food and Agriculture Organization of the United Nations (FAO), in collaboration with the World Health Organization (WHO), have coordinated the prevention and control of the disease and supported eradication efforts in infected countries. Despite these efforts, the disease persists in some regions of the world, while other countries are at risk.

Enforcement of a control strategy based only on sanitary measures, comprising increased biosecurity and culling of animals that are infected or suspected of being infected, has proven to be insufficient to avoid the spread of infection in certain countries. When early detection and rapid response are not adequately implemented, mass depopulation not only raises serious ethical questions for the general public but is also costly and results in economic losses for the owners of the animals, governments and other stakeholders.

The use of vaccines in the current crisis has been limited, owing to logistical difficulties in implementing vaccination programmes in rural areas and the cost and insufficient availability of high-quality vaccine, especially in developing countries and those with economies in transition. Use of some vaccines has been limited by the difficulty of differentiating infected from uninfected animals after vaccination when appropriate. Vaccination campaigns and virus circulation must be monitored in order to prevent spread of the disease through the trade or movement of apparently uninfected animals, their products or the boxes and crates in which they are transported. One of the main concerns of importing countries is that these measures are not fully implemented, and export bans have often been imposed on countries that enforce a vaccination policy.

The OIE and FAO recommend use of vaccination in certain situations, as part of an overall integrated strategy to control the disease. With a clearly defined exit strategy, using the DIVA ('differentiating infected from vaccinated animals') approach or frequent monitoring of sentinel birds, vaccination has successfully controlled or prevented the disease in several situations. Nevertheless, ensuring vaccine quality and their appropriate use is a significant issue in many countries and should form part of the national intervention strategies of countries at risk.

The OIE and FAO considered that it was timely to convene the best-known experts in the field to address global guidelines for vaccination with regard to international standards, regulations and the implementation of programmes. This scientific conference on vaccination, organized by the OIE, FAO and the Istituto Zooprofilattico Sperimentale delle Venezie and supported by the European Commission, was an opportunity to review current methods and recent experiences in the use of vaccination to control and prevent losses due to avian influenza and to discuss appropriate decision-making for implementation of a vaccination strategy.

Dodet B and the Scientific & Technical Department of the OIE (eds): Vaccination: A Tool for the Control of Avian Influenza. Dev Biol (Basel). Basel, Karger, 2007, vol 130, p 1.

SESSION I

Setting the Scene

Chairperson: *I. Capua*, IZSV, Italy

Dodet B and the Scientific & Technical Department of the OIE (eds): Vaccination: A Tool for the Control of Avian Influenza. Dev Biol (Basel). Basel, Karger, 2007, vol 130, pp 3-5.

Highly Pathogenic Avian Influenza: an Update

K. Ben Jebara

Head, Animal Health Information Department, World Organisation for Animal Health (OIE), Paris, France

Key words: Avian influenza, HPAI, H5N1

Highly pathogenic avian influenza (HPAI) virus subtype H5N1 has begun to re-emerge in some countries that had already eradicated the disease. The H5N1 HPAI epizootic that started in South-East Asia at the end of 2003 and remained confined to this region in 2004, spread to other regions and continents in 2005 and 2006. No new countries had been affected in early 2007.

In 2006, 47 countries (8 in Africa, 15 in Asia and 24 in Europe) reported HPAI outbreaks of disease due to the Asian strain of H5N1 in poultry or wild birds. In Europe, the majority of confirmed cases involved wild birds. The very cold winter that occurred in central Europe in early 2006 is thought to have resulted in the movement of wild birds southwards (to Italy, the Balkan region and Greece) and to have been responsible for the cases of HPAI identified there. Most of the affected countries succeeded in eradicating the disease in 2006; however, in some countries, such as Egypt, Indonesia and Nigeria, and to a certain extent China, the disease became endemic and a large number of outbreaks were not reported.

In November 2006, the Republic of Korea reported the re-occurrence of HPAI virus subtype H5N1, the previous reported outbreak having been in March 2004. Viet Nam reported the re-occurrence of H5N1 HPAI in December 2006, 5 months after the previous reported outbreak, in August 2006, and used blanket vaccination against HPAI to control the disease. The re-occurrence is for the time being limited to the extreme south of the country, and the total number of reported outbreaks appears to be more limited than those reported in 2004 and 2005. Thailand reported the re-occurrence of H5N1 HPAI in January 2007, the first reported outbreaks in the country since 2 August 2006. The first occurrence of the disease in this country was in January 2004, and it took almost 32 months to eradicate. Thailand uses stamping-out as its strategy to eradicate the disease, and vaccination is prohibited. Intensive surveillance is organized regularly. In early 2007, Japan reported outbreaks of H5N1

HPAI in Miyasaki and Okojama, in the southern part of the country. The previous occurrence of the disease was in March 2004. As in Thailand, a stamping-out strategy is used to control the disease, and vaccination is prohibited.

Hungary reported re-occurrence of HPAI in January 2007, in two flocks of geese in Csongrad County. The first consisted of 3355 geese in a commercial unit in Szentes-Lapistó, Szentes, and the second of 9386 geese in Derekegyház-Ördöngös, Szentes. The previous reported outbreak in the country was in June 2006. In late January 2007, the United Kingdom reported the re-occurrence of HPAI, in a turkey meat production plant in Upper Holton, Suffolk, England. Virological examination revealed the virus to be of Asian lineage, and molecular genetics studies revealed that the nucleotide sequence of the haemagglutinin gene, one of eight genes, was identical to that of the isolate of H5N1 HPAI from the outbreak in domestic geese in Hungary. The source of introduction of the disease into the affected farm is not yet known, and investigations are in progress. The previous occurrence of H5N1 HPAI reported by the United Kingdom was in March 2006, when a single case was confirmed in a wild whooper swan found dead at Anstruther in Scotland. No domestic poultry were affected at that time.

In February 2007, Turkey reported the re-occurrence of H5N1 HPAI in Batman and Dyarbakir, in the eastern part of the country. The previous occurrence in Turkey was in March 2006. In early February 2007, Pakistan reported re-occurrence of the disease in backyard poultry in North-West Frontier Province, not far from the border with China. The previous reported outbreak was in July 2006. The Lao People's Democratic Republic reported the re-occurrence of HPAI in early February 2007, nearly 7 months after the previous reported outbreak, in July 2006.

In February 2007, the Russian Federation reported three outbreaks of H5N1 HPAI in Krasnodarskiy Kray, near the Black Sea, in native chickens and traditionally raised ducks, geese and turkey cocks. Further outbreaks were reported in the Moskovskaya region, near Moscow. The source of infection is thought to have been birds in a live-bird market in Sadovod, near Moscow, as birds bought at this market had been introduced into the affected backyard flocks. These were the first reported outbreak in the Russian Federation since August 2006. Vaccination is permitted in the country as control measure.

As part of its active surveillance programme on avian influenza, Hong Kong (China) has reported cases of H5N1 HPAI in dead wild birds (*Lonchura punctulata*) that are distributed throughout southern China (Yunnan, Guangxi, Fujian and Hainan), Taiwan China, northern Thailand, the Lao People's Democratic Republic, Cambodia and Viet Nam. An intensive surveillance system is in place on all poultry farms and in other locations in Hong Kong. No evidence of the disease has been found in domestic birds.

In 2006, many countries eradicated the disease in poultry or reported that the disease had not been identified in wild birds. The reports on the re-occurrence of H5N1 HPAI outbreaks in several previously affected countries indicate that most of these countries are now better prepared for early detection of and rapid response to new outbreaks of the disease. Most veterinary services are now ready to tackle the disease when it occurs. A few countries that have been affected for several years are still having difficulty in bringing the disease under control, and the endemic nature of the disease in these countries constitutes a permanent source of potential contamination for humans; it could also be a source of contamination for other countries, through illegal movement of animals, for example.

H5N1 HPAI in animals remains a threat to public health. Nigeria recently confirmed its first human fatality due to H5N1 HPAI. Egypt has confirmed 22 human cases, 13 of which were fatal, and Indonesia and China each confirmed one fatal human case in 2006.

Dr. Karim Ben Jebara, World Organisation for Animal Health (OIE), 12 rue de Prony, 75017 Paris, France
E-mail: k.benjebara@oie.int

Dodet B and the Scientific & Technical Department of the OIE (eds): Vaccination: A Tool for the Control of Avian Influenza. Dev Biol (Basel). Basel, Karger, 2007, vol 130, pp 7-12.

Disease Intelligence for Highly Pathogenic Avian Influenza

J. Domenech[1], J. Slingenbergh[1], V. Martin[1], A. McLeod[1], J. Lubroth[1], L.D. Sims[2]

1 Food and Agriculture Organization of the United Nations, Rome, Italy

2 Asia Pacific Veterinary Information Services, Queensland, Australia

Key words: HPAI, influenza, risk assessment, poultry farming

Summary: A comprehensive approach to highly pathogenic avian influenza (HPAI) is crucial for identifying all the factors that contribute to its emergence, spread and persistence. Epidemiological understanding makes it possible to predict the evolution of the virus and to prevent and control the socioeconomic, environmental, institutional and policy consequences. At FAO, risk assessment and intelligence with regard to HPAI are based on lessons learnt from assisting countries to design strategies and on implementation of technical assistance programmes, which reveal important elements, such as the roles of ducks, live-bird markets and trade. Wild birds were found to contribute, by transporting the H5N1 virus over long distances. The contributions of different poultry farming systems and market chains in the epidemiology of HPAI are well recognized; however, the respective roles of smallholder systems and commercial farms are unclear. FAO considers that smallholders will continue to be an important factor and should be taken into account in control and prevention programmes. Changes in poultry farming are essentially driven by the private sector and market forces and could have negative consequences on the livelihoods of smallholders and on ecologically balanced production systems and agricultural biodiversity. Biosecurity can, however, be improved at the level of farms and markets. Institutional factors, such as the capacity of animal health systems to deliver control programmes, are also important, requiring strengthening and innovation in risk analysis and management.

Tools and Methods

The tools and methods of disease intelligence are needed to address the epidemiology and ecology of avian influenza and its socioeconomic, institutional and policy aspects. Such tools have been designed by two other organizations that are active in animal health, including zoonotic diseases, namely the World Organisation for Animal Health (OIE) and the World Health Organization (WHO).

Rumour tracking allows verification of information on outbreaks from various official sources, including FAO country representatives and field officers, the Global Information and Early Warning System on Food and Agriculture, the Global Public Health Intelligence Network and the Programme for Monitoring of Emerging Diseases. Information systems, such as the World Animal Health Information System of OIE and the Transboundary Animal Disease Information System of FAO, provide official data on animal health status and also unofficial information on animal populations, the movement of animals, products and humans, trade and market chains, climate, land use, wild bird migration routes and natural and man-made disasters.

These layers of information, which are available in FAO statistical data systems (PriceSTAT, TradeSTAT, ProdSTAT, ResourceSTAT and the Global Livestock Production and Health Atlas), are used for epidemiological analysis, modelling and prediction. The FAO-OIE-WHO Global Warning System is a platform set up at international level to monitor global disease evolution and to issue warnings.

Disease tracking, data analysis and disease intelligence are essential for understanding the epidemiology of diseases, health situations and trends. This understanding will allow better-targeted surveillance, prediction, awareness and reporting, including official reporting to the OIE, and the design of the best possible strategies to prevent and control disease.

Emergence of Highly Pathogenic Avian Influenza

HPAI is a zoonotic disease and, like many other pathogens that can shift from animals to humans, its emergence might have been triggered by a combination of human demography, world agricultural dynamics and other factors in global change. The incidence of HPAI has been rising for several decades, coinciding with the rapid growth of the world poultry industry. The switch from low- to highly pathogenic avian influenza appears to take place with the carriage by a wild bird of a virus of low pathogenicity (LPAI) into a poultry holding, where it may circulate without becoming more pathogenic. Repeated exposure may enhance the probability of successful introduction and initial establishment of the virus. So far, the subtypes H5 and H7 have been found to switch to HPAI, but H9 is widespread in Asian poultry and may one day also become highly pathogenic [1].

The number of countries reporting HPAI has increased steadily since the 1980s. H5N1 HPAI virus was first reported in 1996, in domestic waterfowl in Guangdong Province in China. Hong Kong SAR was the first area to experience human deaths due to H5N1 HPAI [2], in 1997. Since then, the virus has continued to circulate among domestic waterfowl in China and, following the emergence of genotypes Z and Z+ in 2003, began to cause human deaths in mainland China.

Spread of Highly Pathogenic Avian Influenza

The spread of H5N1 HPAI in poultry across the subcontinent began in 2003, involving Indonesia and the Republic of Korea, but became manifest in early 2004, when it was found in countries across South-East and eastern Asia [3]. Human cases of avian influenza were first detected in Viet Nam and Thailand, and more cases were detected later elsewhere.

It soon became apparent that the circulation of H5N1 virus in poultry was the main source of human infection. Most cases of infection occurred in persons handling sick or dead birds in their backyards, in live-bird markets or in the kitchen. Chicken are the most numerous poultry species [4] and are highly susceptible to H5N1 HPAI. Broilers continue to be the main source of human H5N1 infection. The consumption of duck, particularly on the occasion of the Chinese lunar New Year, was initially believed to contribute to human infection, but this hypothesis was later discarded, as consumption of poultry is usually not responsible for human infections; nevertheless, a number of mammals that eat bird carcasses and birds of prey became infected with H5N1 virus.

The disease in both poultry and humans appears to be seasonal, and the seasonality of human infection was found to be associated with the seasonal flare-up of disease in poultry [5]. Another factor is the decreased ambient temperatures and increased humidity during winter, which reduce the rate of decay of H5N1 virus outside the avian host and may enhance avian-to-human transmission. The increase in outbreaks of H5N1 HPAI in poultry during winter has been seen not only in Asia but also in Europe and Africa. The determinants of seasonality are not, however, identical in all ecopathological and geographical settings. In Asia, the congregation of large populations of domestic ducks in wetlands during autumn, following the monsoon rice harvest, may also create H5N1 HPAI hot spots.

Duck and Rice Farming Systems and Highly Pathogenic Avian Influenza

FAO has coordinated a number of studies on the role of free-range ducks in the spread and persistence of HPAI. The results show that areas with year-round rice production in wetlands, where the local hydrology supports irrigated rice cropping, also support egg production by ducks grazing in post-harvest rice paddies throughout the year [6]. The rice harvest associated with the monsoon season provides the bulk of the total rice production and enables the production of duck meat from September to January, right up to the Chinese New Year. Layer ducks produce eggs for consumers and for the synchronized release of ducklings for meat production. The hatching of eggs and raising of ducklings are carefully planned for the release of the ducklings into post-harvest rice paddies, where feed is abundant after the monsoon rice harvest.

The release of large numbers of ducklings into rice fields was found to coincide with epidemic waves of H5N1 HPAI in the central plains of Thailand and in the Mekong delta of Viet Nam. Free-range ducks also have an important role elsewhere in Asia. The temporospatial pattern of rice harvesting determines duck husbandry and thus modulates the persistence of H5N1 HPAI virus, at least in areas with large duck populations. Rice harvests can be monitored with satellites in order to predict when and where the risk for HPAI emergence is highest [7]. While more analysis is needed, this tool might be of practical use in early warning systems.

Other Risk Factors for Highly Pathogenic Avian Influenza H5N1

The subcontinental spread of H5N1 HPAI genotype Z in late 2003 and early 2004 probably occurred mainly through trade and traffic of chickens, which might also have involved commercial circuits. While large-scale poultry factories are relatively biosecure, commercial poultry chains can be taken by surprise, and industrial plants incurred relatively heavy losses during the first waves of the epidemic, due not only to imposed trade restrictions but also to clinical disease and mortality and to culling.

The H5N1 virus established itself rapidly in live-bird markets, also infecting backyard and open duck farming systems. Its persistence in poultry faeces and contamination of fomites have proven critical to viral traffic in the contact network. H5N1 HPAI viruses themselves are of variable pathogenicity and also show marked differences in disease severity by poultry species: while chicken and other terrestrial poultry species, including quails and turkeys, are highly susceptible to H5N1 viruses, domestic waterfowl show variable degrees of disease resistance.

Since 2001, the prevalence of H5N1 virus in ducks and geese in China has increased [5,8,9]. It is possible that the high pathogenicity of H5N1 viruses in chicken leads to rapid spread but perhaps not to virus persistence, at least in the absence of a reservoir; however, the presence of birds that are susceptible and resistant to H5N1 HPAI, such as ducks and chicken, poultry and wild birds or a mix of susceptible and resistant wild birds, would facilitate both virus spread and persistence. Following the major episode of deaths due to H5N1 HPAI among bar-headed geese in the spring of 2005 in Qinghai Lake in China, the same virus was isolated in the summer of 2005 in Kazakhstan, Mongolia and the Russian Federation [10]. The dispersal from east to west, from China to Siberia and from there to the Caspian Sea, Black Sea and the Mediterranean basin, is consistent with vectoring of the virus by migratory birds. Poultry arguably enhanced this process, supporting local redistribution of the virus. Eventually, a Europe–Middle East–Africa H5N1 clade evolved.

While poultry trade and traffic are generally the most important force behind the spread of H5N1 virus, wild birds continue to support its spread over long distances. Studies initiated by FAO to clarify the precise role of wild birds in the epidemiology of HPAI indicate that H5N1 HPAI may also be carried by migratory birds in sub-Saharan Africa. Studies in Asia, with transmitters mounted on swans migrating after the 2006 summer breeding from Mongolia, revealed that the migration routes of individual birds are highly variable. A study of the land use pattern in locations selected by birds for staging and overwintering showed that the risk factors vary from country to country and even from year to year.

It is impossible to identify the countries at highest risk. Densely populated, advanced developing countries with urban populations that buy large numbers of broilers from live-bird markets daily are at high risk, particularly when neighbouring countries already have the infection. Live-bird markets are thus important nodes in the viral traffic network. The production sector of any country comprises four distinct subsectors, as defined by FAO: industrial poultry plants, which are fully integrated vertically (subsector 1); large-scale commercial holdings, which are not fully integrated (subsector 2); medium-sized holdings and associated marketing networks (subsector 3); and backyard or village poultry farms (subsector 4). Depending on the specific set of circumstances and the stage of the epidemic, all these subsectors may play a role. Still, most virus circulation is believed to occur in subsectors 3 and 4. Large domestic duck populations in open systems in particular support persistence of the virus. Seasonal release of ducklings can trigger epidemic waves, but differently in different latitudes. The presence of the virus in neighbouring countries, live-bird markets, mixed poultry production systems, mixed poultry species, contacts with migratory birds, urban concentration and the efficacy of public and veterinary services collectively determine whether a country will become infected with H5N1

HPAI. Hence, in high-risk countries, the probable socioeconomic impact of the disease and of its control and the prospects for successful control can be reasonably well predicted.

Highly Pathogenic Avian Influenza beyond the Veterinary Realm

A high level of socioeconomic development is key to successful control and prevention of HPAI infection. A decision to invest in biosecurity is usually taken by individual producers in order to protect the health of their animals and to produce more effectively, as investment in animal health protection always results in an incremental increase in production. Farmers who invest in medicines, vaccines, cages, sheds, fences and other forms of biosecurity will be paid back in improved production. Farmers who cannot engage in economies of scale, the main prerequisite for reducing the cost of poultry production, are also unable to pay a high price for biosecurity. Smallholder poultry producers instead select disease- or parasite-resistant birds that are good scavengers and adapt to local circumstances.

Agrobiodiversity is most frequent in traditional husbandry systems with poor market access. Poultry may not yield much income or even food but are nevertheless key to sustaining livelihoods. Socioeconomic analyses undertaken by FAO revealed that rural societies in developing countries are often severely hit by HPAI, not so much in terms of food security but because poultry are generally very important for their livelihood [11]. This finding indicates that, in situations in which the virus has become established in poultry, aggressive culling to contain spread of the virus might be ineffective or counterproductive and would be immoral when there is no compensation, particularly when the outcome of culling on virus circulation is unpredictable. In these situations, a comprehensive approach is needed, and incorporating vaccination into the package might well be an efficient, viable option.

FAO Risk Assessment: The Big Picture

The HPAI risk assessment undertaken by FAO incorporates various socioeconomic, environmental, institutional and policy considerations. The global perspective studies focus on how agricultural landscapes are transformed over time [12,13]. Predictions show that by 2030 developing countries will still count a rural population of 3.5 billion people, comprising farmers, their families and rural village communities, many of which will continue to rely in one way or another on poultry husbandry for their livelihood. Poor countries in Asia and Africa have relatively large rural populations. Disease control and prevention programmes will have to take this into account.

Changes in poultry production are essentially driven by the private sector and market forces, which can have negative consequences on the livelihoods of smallholders and on ecologically balanced production systems and agricultural biodiversity. Biosecurity can, however, be improved at the level of farms and markets. Institutional factors, such as national animal health systems, including public veterinary services, are key to area-wide disease prevention and control. Risky practices, such as major live-bird trade and traffic, are a public concern, as is the presence of industrial plants and smallholders around urban centres. Combinations of the FAO subsectors might result in conflicting biosecurity regimes. Hence, it is necessary to address the full picture, expanding risk assessment as required for adequate, comprehensive risk management, with consideration of animal health, public health, rural livelihoods and sustainable agricultural development [14]. This is a major challenge, as it involves upgrading animal health systems worldwide.

References

1 Alexander DJ: Summary of avian influenza activity in Europe, Asia, Africa and Australasia, 2002-2006. Avian Dis 2006;51:161-166.

2 Shortridge KF, Zhou NN, Guan Y, Gao P, Ito T, Kawaoka Y, Kodihalli S, Krauss S, Markwell D, Murti KG, Norwood M, Senne D, Sims L, Takada A, Webster RG: Characterization of avian H5N1 influenza viruses from poultry in Hong Kong. Virology 1998;252:331-342.

3 Martin V, Sims L, Lubroth J, Pfeiffer D, Slingenbergh J, Domenech J: Epidemiology and ecology of highly pathogenic avian influenza with particular emphasis on South East Asia. Dev Biol (Basel) 2006;124:23-36.

4 FAO: FAOSTAT, 2006: http://faostat.fao.org/site/409/default.aspx.

5 Li KS,Guan Y, Wang J, Smith GJ, Xu KM, Duan L, Rahardjo AP, Puthavathana P, Buranathai C, Nguyen TD, Estoepangestie AT, Chaisingh A, Auewarakul P, Long HT, Hanh NT, Webby RJ, Poon LL, Chen H, Shortridge KF, Yuen KY, Webster RG, Peiris JS: Genesis of a highly pathogenic and potentially pandemic H5N1 influenza virus in eastern Asia. Nature 2004;430:209-213.

6 Gilbert M, Chaitaweesub P, Parakamawongsa T, Premashthira S, Tiensin T, Kalpravidh W, Wagner H, Slingenbergh J: Free-grazing ducks and highly pathogenic avian influenza, Thailand. Emerg Infect Dis 2006;12:227-234.

7 Xiao X et al.: Remote sensing, ecological variables and wild bird migration related to outbreaks of highly pathogenic H5N1 bird flu. J Wildl Dis 2007; in press.

8 Chen H, Deng G, Li Z, Tin G, Li Y, Jiao P, Zhang L, Liu Z, Webster RG, Yu K: The evolution of H5N1 influenza viruses in ducks in southern China. Proc Natl Acad Sci USA 2004;101:10452-10457.

9 Hulse-Post D, Sturm-Ramirez KM, Humberd J, Seiler P, Govorkova EA, Krauss S, Scholtissek C, Puthavathana P, Buranathai C, Nguyen TD, Long HT, Naipospos TSP, Guan Y, Peiris JSM, Webster RG: Role of domestic ducks in the propagation and biological evolution of highly pathogenic H5N1 influenza viruses in Asia. Proc Natl Acad Sci USA 2005;102:10682-10687.

10 Liu J, Xiao H, Lei F, Zhu Q, Qin K, Zhang XW, Zhaing XI, Dhao D, Wang G, Feng Y, Ma J, Liu W, Wang J, Gao F: Highly pathogenic H5N1 influenza virus infection in migratory birds. Science 2005, 309:1206.

11 Rushton J, Viscarra R, Guerne-Bleich E, Mcleod A: Impact of avian influenza outbreaks in the poultry sectors of five south east Asian countries (Cambodia, Indonesia, Lao PDR, Thailand, Viet Nam) outbreak costs, responses and potential long term control. World Poultry Sci J 2005;24:491-514.

12 Bruinsma J: World Agriculture: Towards 2015/2030: An FAO Perspective. London, Earthscan Publications, 2003.

13 FAO: World agriculture: towards 2030/2050, prospects for food, nutrition, agriculture and major commodity groups, interim report. Rome, Food and Agriculture Organization of the United Nations, 2006.

14 FAO, OIE: A global Strategy for the Progressive Control of Highly Pathogenic Avian Influenza (HPAI). Rome, Food and Agriculture Organization of the United Nations, 2007.

Dr. Jan Slingenbergh, FAO (AGAH), Viale delle Terme di Caracalla, 00153 Rome, Italy
E-mail: jan.slingenbergh@fao.org

Dodet B and the Scientific & Technical Department of the OIE (eds): Vaccination: A Tool for the Control of Avian Influenza. Dev Biol (Basel). Basel, Karger, 2007, vol 130, pp 13-21.

Control Strategies for Highly Pathogenic Avian Influenza: a Global Perspective

J. Lubroth

Emergency Prevention System for Transboundary Animal Pests and Plant Diseases, Animal Health Service, Animal Production and Health Division, Food and Agriculture Organization of the United Nations, Rome, Italy

Key words: HPAI, H5N1, avian influenza, control strategies

Summary: Comprehensive programmes for the prevention, detection and control of highly pathogenic avian influenza (HPAI) require a national dimension and relevant national legislation in which veterinary services can conduct surveillance, competent diagnosis and rapid response. Avian influenza was controlled and prevented by vaccination long before the current H5N1 crisis. The use of vaccine cannot be separated from other essential elements of a vaccination campaign, which include education in poultry production practices, such as hygiene, all in–all out production concepts, separation of species, biosecurity (bio-exclusion to keep the disease out and biocontainment to keep the disease from spreading once suspected or detected), competence in giving the vaccine and the role of vaccination teams, post-vaccination monitoring to ensure efficacy and to detect the circulation of wild-type virus, surveillance and buffer zones in outbreak areas, and performance indicators to determine when vaccination can cease. Reporting of disease can be improved through well-structured, adequately financed veterinary services and also by fair compensation for producers who suffer financial loss. A rapid response to suspected cases of HPAI should be ensured in simulation exercises involving various sectors of the food production and marketing chain, policy-makers, official veterinary structures and other government personnel. As for other transboundary animal diseases, national approaches must be part of a regional strategy and regional networks for cooperation and information sharing, which in turn reflect global policies and international standards, such as the quality of vaccines, reporting obligations, humane interventions, cleaning and disinfection methods, restocking times, monitoring and safe trade.

INTRODUCTION

The spread of highly pathogenic avian influenza (HPAI) has usually been controlled by surveillance, reporting, detection and response by government veterinary services, and foci of infection have been eliminated by culling diseased or potentially exposed flocks [1-4]. In some instances, similar actions have been taken after the detection of less virulent strains of avian influenza virus, at times with vaccination of poultry stock [2,5]. With the emergence of H5N1 HPAI viruses in Asia in the late 1990s and their spread across Asia, Africa and Europe between 2003 and 2006, causing huge losses in poultry production farms and disruption of people's livelihoods, vaccination has also been considered important in prevention and control in numerous countries, supported by international organizations if accompanied by ancillary measures of equal or greater importance.

Requirements for Global Control of Highly Pathogenic Avian Influenza

Good farming practices, education and capacity-building

The use of vaccine cannot be seen in isolation from other essential elements in a prevention, control or vaccination campaign. These include education in good poultry production practices such as farm or household hygiene, all in–all out production concepts, separation of species, biosecurity (bio-exclusion to keep the disease out; biocontainment to keep the disease from spreading once suspected or detected) and well managed and resourced extension services of the public and private sectors. At the technical professional level, veterinary curricula should encompass not only physiology and medicine but also flock health and production and regulatory and public health matters.

National, regional and international dimensions

As for other transboundary animal diseases, national approaches must be part of any regional strategy, which in turn should reflect global policies and standards, such as the quality of vaccines, reporting obligations, humane interventions, cleaning and disinfection in an environmentally safe manner, the principles and needs for restocking, monitoring and promotion of safe trade [6,7].

Essential in the development of a national plan for prevention and control of HPAI is the notion of a robust partnership with the widest range of stakeholders or interested parties (producers, transport companies, meat packers, regulatory personnel and other public servants), so that individual interests can be expressed and a common understanding of national needs achieved [3]. In this environment, immediate and longer-term measures can be considered through a programmatic approach to preventing, detecting and tackling HPAI in domestic poultry [6,7].

From a national perspective, the key elements in a strategy to prevent, control, eliminate or eradicate HPAI viruses include: (i) legislation that facilitates rapid intervention, quarantine inspection and regulatory control, with immediate access to contingency funds for a declared emergency; (ii) an emergency management and response structure for disasters (i.e. HPAI); (iii) risk analyses with programmed surveillance and targeted epidemiological approaches; (iv) proficient veterinary diagnostic laboratories; (v) regular and maintained inspection, appropriate importation and quarantine regimes, border control and movement management; (vi) education, awareness and communication; (vii) rehabilitation or restructuring programmes for various sectors to ensure good farming practices; (viii) emergency preparedness and contingency planning, with rehearsed field exercises; and (ix) a research agenda for improvement of risk analysis, vaccines and their use, epidemiological methods or improved understanding of ecological factors that affect disease occurrence, including virological, diagnostic, wildlife interactions, virus and host factors, poultry and vaccine, epidemiological or socioeconomic issues in a national or subnational context. Improved reporting of disease requires well-structured, adequately financed veterinary services and a just means of compensation to producers and families who suffer losses. Rapid response to suspected cases of HPAI should be practised through field simulation exercises involving various sectors of the food production and marketing chain, policy-makers, private and official veterinary structures and other government personnel [7].

The same elements should be present at regional and international levels, to ensure networks in countries or in economic market groupings, to stimulate horizontal information-sharing and building of trust across borders and partners. Similar thematic networks are also important, whereby reference laboratory personnel, socioeconomic experts and wildlife specialists can share their experiences with national and regional entities [6-8].

The following guiding principles were used by FAO and the OIE in formulating a global strategy for the control of HPAI, which could be adapted to the national context [6,7]:

- Commitment: The prevention, control and elimination of HPAI from the domestic poultry sector are for the global public good, requiring strong national, regional and international commitment at political, financial and technical levels.
- Multidisciplinarity and broad collaboration: HPAI control programmes require multidisciplinary approaches integrating technical, social, financial, political, policy and regulatory experts.
- Adaptability and knowledge base: The strategy must be flexible and should incorporate new information and technology as they become available and are tested or validated.
- Sensitivity to people's livelihoods: The global strategy takes into account the importance of poultry to the livelihoods of the rural and urban poor, who are the most vulnerable and often the most severely affected.
- Economic sustainability: The strategy encourages equitable growth of the poultry sector through a combination of activities that benefit the poor and stimulate market-based commercial growth.

Surveillance, reporting and effective response

Progressive control requires tackling the disease at source, which, for HPAI, is domestic poultry. Clinical and pathological findings of HPAI in certain species of poultry, such as turkeys, chickens and quail, should be sufficient to raise an alarm to producers, veterinarians and veterinary authorities, and a thorough epidemiological investigation should be carried out, samples taken and a differential diagnosis performed to identify the cause. Should the findings be of epidemiological significance or if reporting to national authorities is obligatory, this must be done immediately without political or trade-related pressures. Surveillance should be structured to incorporate risk-based approaches but also allow routine inspection and submission of samples in a programmed monitoring scheme.

Although epidemiological studies suggest that wild birds probably play a role in the transmission of avian influenza viruses to domestic poultry and vice versa [2,9-14], the sustained capacity of wild birds to carry an HPAI virus such as H5N1 has not been demonstrated [12,15]. A known avian influenza virus in the wild bird population could not be eradicated, nor should governments or producers divert valuable resources to this effort.

After detection of an HPAI virus, a rapid, effective response entails 'standstill' orders, humane culling, proper disposal of carcasses by burial, burning, rendering or composting, cleaning and disinfection, and a period during which susceptible poultry are not on the premises [3]. These six actions (standstill, culling, disposal, cleaning, disinfection and vacancy) remain the cornerstone of an effective response if the virus has been detected early enough. The availability of a compensation fund is critical for early reporting and detection, and a well-practised team of responders is critical to decrease the likelihood of disease spread [4].

Regional and global commitment and investment to study the ecology of avian influenza viruses in their natural cycles and to further understand wild bird hosts would lead to early-warning systems if the viruses are characterized in parallel with viruses obtained from poultry. The combination of field studies with experimental work on different avian and mammalian hosts would allow better understanding of risks, pathogenesis, maintenance reservoirs and the efficacy of vaccines to protect species in at-risk aviaries and other valuable collections [2,11,16,17].

Targeting the disease at source

One of the key activities of FAO's Emergency Prevention System for Transboundary Animal and Plant Pests and Diseases (EMPRES) is early warning of disease occurrence and forecasts of possible disease spread. To promote prevention as a cost-effective approach to mitigation of disease risk or progressive control, disease control and eradication campaigns should focus on the origin of infection, transmission and disease. Targeted approaches to protect susceptible hosts from infection include limiting the movement of potentially amplifying hosts, modifying the environment or behaviour that accentuates the risk for infection and concentrating activities in endemic zones rather than in those that are free of disease. Although this approach makes sense-medically and financially-it is rarely practised. In the case of H5N1 HPAI, the international and regional strategy was to generate national commitment and financial assistance for countries in Asia before the disease spread to other countries and continents. Insufficient commitment from several countries or emphasis on non-amplifying or reservoir hosts detracted from activities directed at the poultry source, where the risk for infection was highest, to other avian and mammalian species (including humans); it also resulted in insufficient control of animal movement, markets and product trade.

In the case of H5N1 HPAI, the source of infection is predominantly the smallholder poultry sector or the domestic duck population [14,17]. Although wild birds are known reservoirs of numerous avian influenza viruses, the current global emphasis is to enhance biosecurity by promoting safe trade and husbandry and keeping wild birds away from poultry. In countries with large duck populations dispersed among gallinaceous species, the national strategies and global recommendations for disease control include changes in domestic duck farming to separate domestic ducks from terrestrial poultry and wild birds, strategic culling of domestic ducks among which HPAI virus is found and progressive enhancement of flock immunity by systematic vaccination campaigns to reduce the viral load and virus shedding, where vaccine use is not banned [3,17]. In industrial poultry farming, preventing and controlling the disease by reducing virus circulation in large-scale breeder units and medium-to-small commercial units is far more feasible in the short and medium term. Vaccinating day-old chicks and young goslings in hatcheries has technical merit and could be an important intervention, as the animals are concentrated and vaccination is relatively easy. Mapping hatcheries (of which there may be 100 or more in a medium-sized country) and delivering vaccine are logistically difficult, but less so than achieving the same coverage by field, farm or household visits.

There is no doubt that, for a virus such as H5N1, elimination of the source from backyard poultry will be arduous and long, especially in countries with weak veterinary administrations, limited financial resources, no compensation strategy and poor governance by leaders and decision-makers.

Vaccination as a response

As stated by others, vaccination alone is insufficient to control and eradicate an incursion of HPAI. In addition, if a decision has been taken to use vaccine (imported or manufactured nationally), it must meet or exceed international standards for potency, efficacy and safety [6,18]. Competence in giving the vaccine is also required, and the responsibility of vaccination teams to meet biosecurity safety criteria must be ensured [3].

The decision to include vaccination as part of an HPAI control and eradication campaign should be carefully evaluated case by case, and may rest on when the disease was first detected, how far and at which speed it has spread, and the infrastructure and finances available to administer the vaccine strategically and operationally. Post-vaccination monitoring is required to ensure or improve efficacy, and surveillance must be maintained for persistence of wild-type virus [6]. Should virus circulation be documented, producers and regulatory authorities must share the responsibility for faults in response measures and take corrective action.

It is difficult but necessary to decide on ceasing vaccination when control measures have been effective for some time. An exit strategy must be decided upon after consideration of several factors and indicators for the absence of circulation of HPAI virus and the activities undertaken by industry, farmers and veterinary regulatory officials. The factors to be considered are the absence of avian influenza virus in clinical cases suspected to be caused by syndromes consistent with possible HPAI infection in poultry (and in instances of zoonotic avian influenza virus with no human illnesses reported), no seroconversion or virus detection in sentinel birds within vaccinated flocks, no serological conversion to N1S [19], no seroconversion to N-antigens representative of the wild-type virus that caused HPAI outbreaks in which heterologous or recombinant vaccines were used [2,20], vaccine coverage, knowledge of marketing flows and structures (see below) and other criteria established by consultation with stakeholders. The elements and activities required to determine whether vaccine use should be suspended include the ability of the surveillance system to detect infection or disease in the field and laboratory and the response capability, such as the status of neighbouring countries and trading partners and the ability to apply appropriate surveillance and buffer zones in outbreak areas. Maintenance of a certain number of doses of vaccine should be considered, taking into account poultry numbers and production schemes, risk areas and the status of neighbouring countries.

Marketing systems and responsibilities of veterinary regulatory services

A vital part of an effective response is advance knowledge of existing production and marketing systems, such that trace-forward and trace-back activities can be instituted at once and disease surveillance, awareness and mitigation measures undertaken. As dynamic changes can occur rapidly in poultry production (largely due to the fast growing period between hatching and market weight) and in the financial preferences of producers or sectors, the markets should be studied regularly and often. In addition, the regulatory veterinary services should conduct surveillance and inspection so that ante-mortem and post-mortem examinations guarantee that only wholesome products enter the food chain and slaughter houses meet hygienic requirements. Local market practices and neighbourhood butcheries in a number of countries represent a risk for disease incursion and spread if there is no system for detection or control, but these should at least be registered, proprietors informed of their obligations and responsibilities, and inspections carried out regularly to ensure compliance.

Systems forbidding the return of unsold poultry to their farms of origin and establishing several days a week when poultry or their products are not sold, thus permitting proper cleaning and disinfection, would curtail the risk for spread of disease through marketing channels. Compliance with the system would be ensured by veterinary inspection agencies, including separation of species on marketing days, proper disposal of refuse and proper refrigeration temperatures, where available.

Poultry sectors

Characterization of a national poultry flock into the admittedly blurred four poultry production sectors 1-4 [7] is important. The description should include census, distribution, proportional contribution and market activities to help understand the risks for disease introduction, plan awareness and intervention measures including vaccine needs, socioeconomic studies and provide guidance for improved prevention of transboundary avian diseases, such as HPAI [4,6,14].

Contingency plans and emergency preparedness centres

A contingency plan for an incursion of transboundary animal disease should comprise a strategy and a response. Contingency plans are technical documents to guide the public sector response to an emergency. Critical to the success of a contingency plan and its implementation is the involvement of stakeholders from the private sector, including industry. Early on, a national steering committee should be set up, with key decision-makers and stakeholders, perhaps including national experts, research institutes and nongovernmental organizations, to oversee the plan and its testing in simulation exercises (both as observers and participants). Practised (and updated) contingency plans with a properly staffed and resourced management response centre are indicative of a modern veterinary service [3].

The technical description of a contingency plan should be based on national or subnational realities of animal production, censuses, marketing and trade, linking policy, coordination, personnel and financial resources, and sound analyses. A well-rehearsed contingency plan (i.e. in simulation exercises) undoubtedly improves early response, rapid elimination of disease and prompt recovery. Contingency plans should involve not only official veterinary service personnel but also public health officials (especially for zoonotic diseases such as H5N1 HPAI), environmental and wildlife experts, security forces, financial officers, public works and communication and training specialists [3]. In all cases, decision trees (e.g. case definitions, determining whether to use vaccine, compensation), standard operating procedures (e.g. flow of diagnostic samples, wearing protective equipment, compensation) and succinct descriptions of the duties of all personnel (terms of reference and level of responsibility) should be included.

Once a disease such as HPAI has been detected, an emergency management and response centre can serve as a pivot for decisions about operations, ensure that the activities are coordinated, determine the required activities to be implemented on the basis of information from the field, laboratories and epidemiology units and provide a reliable source of updated information for decision-makers.

Conclusions

The success of disease control is measured at the local level but depends on factors distant from the village farmer or household. Essential areas of investment for concerted action against HPAI, other transboundary animal diseases and disaster and emergency response include a baseline census of poultry populations and a description of poultry and livestock production sectors and commerce; a baseline evaluation of the veterinary services in order to identify gaps; strong legal and institutional frameworks to support the control or prevention of transboundary animal diseases; programmes for active surveillance and monitoring of avian influenza and HPAI, including laboratories, epidemiology, information systems and streamlined reporting; assessments of the socioeconomic impact of the disease, including that of the control strategy itself; and contingency and emergency preparedness plans at national level, in partnership with technical and planning departments and ministries of agriculture, human health, environment and finance to improve capacity for long-term strategic planning and response to emergency situations.

Regionally, the approach is to create strong, efficient regional coordination units and support for regional networks of epidemiology and disease surveillance, diagnosis and information sharing, wildlife and socioeconomic studies, policy development and the promotion of good governance and trust.

The potential global impact of HPAI requires countries to use internationally agreed plans for its prevention and progressive control. The main responsibilities of the international partnership, especially among FAO, OIE and WHO, should be to:

- coordinate subregional networks and regional animal health centres;
- sustain and invest further in the tripartite Global Early Warning System for the emergence of new infectious diseases, including HPAI;
- set up multinational, multidisciplinary teams that could be deployed rapidly to assist countries or regions in times of crisis;
- identify and play a strategic role in coordinating research for improved HPAI control between national institutions and reference centres; and
- advocate for resource mobilization for HPAI prevention, control and eradication through diplomatic, political and donor liaisons.

In the case of zoonotic HPAI or avian influenza viruses, strong collaboration between FAO, OIE and WHO on personal protection, epidemiological risk factors in transmission and food safety will be important [2,16]. Relevant common activities, such as the sharing of information on virus isolates and disease, joint field investigations, epidemiological studies, contingency planning and public communication, are required. An international strategy for HPAI must cover a complex matrix of situations, although success is always measured at the local level. Different approaches are required for the different poultry production sectors, and sensitivity is needed to the cultural nuances of production and marketing. A strategy requires components of prevention and emergency preparedness, detection and early response, rehabilitation and restructuring of an affected or at-risk poultry sector. Trade-whether large-scale and international or local for subsistence-must be taken into account, and small producers and family farms must be protected [7].

In order to improve the prevention or management of serious emerging diseases, the global and national community will require enabling legislation; an emergency management and response structure; risk analysis, surveillance and targeted approaches; a veterinary diagnostic laboratory network; appropriate inspection, importation and quarantine regimes, with border control and movement management; education, awareness and communication; rehabilitation or restructuring programmes to improve farming practices; emergency preparedness and contingency plans; and a research agenda to adapt existing knowledge to local situations, to include national needs and improve understanding of disease dynamics and socioeconomic implications.

Acknowledgements

The contributions of countless colleagues, who since 2004 have participated in the formulation, discussions, analysis, language, description and revision of the FAO/OIE strategy, is poorly acknowledged by the authorship of one individual. The author tacitly acknowledges the contributions of dozens of individuals whose ideas are captured in this synopsis of a very complex problem of national and global concern.

References

1 Otte MJ, Nugent R, McLeod A: Transboundary Animal Diseases: Assessment of Socioeconomic Impacts and Institutional Responses (Livestock Policy Discussion Paper No. 9) Rome, Food and Agriculture Organization of the United Nations, 2004.

2 Capua I, Alexander DJ: The challenge of avian influenza to the veterinary community. Avian Pathol 2006; 35:1-17.

3 Martin V, Forman A, Lubroth J: Preparing for Highly Pathogenic Avian Influenza (FAO Production and Health Manual 3), Rome, Food and Agriculture Organization of the United Nations 2006. http://www.fao.org/docs/eims/upload//200354/HPAI_manual.pdf.

4 McLeod A, Morgan N, Prakash A, Hinrichs J: Economic and Social Impacts of Avian Influenza, Rome, Food and Agriculture Organization of the United Nations, 2006. http://www.fao.org/AG/AGAInfo/subjects/en/health/diseases-cards/cd/documents/Economic-and-social-impacts-of-avian-influenza-Geneva.pdf (accessed 6 April 2007).

5 Swayne DE: Vaccines for list A poultry diseases 2003. Emphasis on avian influenza. Dev Biol 2003,114:201-12.

6 FAO, OIE A Global Strategy for the Progressive Control of Highly Pathogenic Avian Influenza (HPAI). Rome, Food and Agriculture Organization of the United Nations, 2005. http://www.fao.org/docs/eims/upload//210745/Glo_pro_HPAI_oct05_en.

7 Lubroth J, Morzaria S, Thiermann AB: Global strategy for highly pathogenic avian influenza: progressive control and eradication, and post-outbreak recovery. In: Swayne DE, ed. Avian Influenza, Ames, Iowa, Blackwell Publishing 2007; in press.

8 Edwards S: OFFLU network on avian influenza. Emerg Infect Dis 2006;8:1287-1288.

9 Ito T, Okazaki K, Kawaoka Y, Takada A, Webster RG, Kida H: Perpetuation of influenza A viruses in Alaskan waterfowl reservoirs. Arch Virol 1995;140: 1163-72.

10 Webster RG, Bean WJ, Gorman OT, Chambers TM, Kawaoka Y: Evolution and ecology of influenza A viruses. Microbiol Rev 1992;56:152-179.

11 Deogu M, De Marco MA, Donatelli I, Campitelli L, Catelli E: Ecological aspects of influenza A virus circulation in wild birds of the western palearctic. Vet Res Commun 2003;27:101-106.

12 Chen H, Smith GJD, Zhang SY, Qin K, Wang J, Li KS, Webster RG, Peiris JSM, Guan Y: H5N1 virus outbreak in migratory waterfowl. Nature 2005;436:191-192.

13 Gilbert M, Xiao X, Domenech J, Lubroth J, Martin V, Slingenbergh J: Anatidae migration in the western palearctic and spread of highly pathogenic avian influenza H5N1 virus. Emerg Infect Dis 2006;12:1650-1656.

14 Martin V, Sims L, Lubroth J, Pfeiffer D, Slingenbergh J, Domenech J: Epidemiology and ecology of highly pathogenic avian influenza with particular emphasis on South-East Asia. Dev Biol (Basel) 2006, 124:23-36.

15 Munster VJ, Wallensten A, Baas C, Rimmelzwaan GF, Schutten M, Olsen B, Osterhaus ADME, Fouchier RAM: Mallards and highly pathogenic avian influenza ancestral viruses, northern Europe. Emerg Infect Dis 2005;11:1545-1551.

16 Perdue ML, Swayne DE: Public health risk from avian influenza viruses. Avian Dis 2005; 49:317-327.

17 Gilbert M, Chaitaweesub P, Parakamaswonga T, Premashthira S, Tiensin T, Kalpravidh W, Wagner H, Slingenbergh: Free-grazing ducks and highly pathogenic avian influenza, Thailand. Emerg Infect Dis 2006;12:227-234.

18 OIE: Manual of Diagnostic Tests and Vaccines for Terrestrial Animals. 5th Ed., Paris, World Organisation for Animal Health, 2004. http://www.oie.int/eng/publicat/en_tarifs.htm.

19 Tumpey TM, Alvarez R, Swayne DE, Suarez DL: Diagnostic approach for differentiating infected from vaccinated poultry on the basis of antibodies to N1S, the nonstructural protein of infulenza A virus. J Clin Microbiol 2005;43:676-683.

20 Swayne DE, Garcia M, Beck JR, Kinney N, Suarez DL: Protection against diverse highly pathogenic avian influenza viruses in chickens immunized with a recombinant fowl pox vaccine containing an H5 avian influenza haemagglutinin gene insert. Vaccine 2000;18:1088-1095.

Dr. Juan Lubroth, Emergency Prevention System for Transboundary Animal Pests and Plant Diseases (EMPRES), Animal Health Service, Animal Production and Health Division, Food and Agriculture Organization of the United Nations, Viale delle Terme di Caracalla, Rome 00100, Italy
E-mail: juan.lubroth@fao.org

Dodet B and the Scientific & Technical Department of the OIE (eds): Vaccination: A Tool for the Control of Avian Influenza. Dev Biol (Basel). Basel, Karger, 2007, vol 130, pp 23-30.

International Standards and Guidelines for Vaccination of Poultry against Highly Pathogenic Avian Influenza

C. Bruschke, G. Brückner, B. Vallat

World Organisation for Animal Health (OIE), Paris, France

Key words: HPAI, H5N1, influenza, vaccination, guidelines

Summary: The current strain of highly pathogenic avian influenza (HPAI), H5N1, has caused an unprecedented situation, spreading over three continents, with severe economic and social consequences. The strategy of the World Organisation for Animal Health (OIE) focuses on the following key actions: early warning, early detection, rapid confirmation of suspected cases, rapid response and rapid and transparent notification. Vaccination is one means that can be used to control the virus. During the current H5N1 outbreak, the OIE received many requests from member countries for guidance in deciding whether to vaccinate and in the design of vaccination programmes. The OIE has published a general information document on vaccination against avian influenza and a document giving guidelines for decision-making, including a checklist of essentials for establishing a vaccination programme.

INTRODUCTION

Avian influenza viruses can be divided into low- and highly pathogenic strains. The low-pathogenicity strains are commonly found in wild waterfowl, and outbreaks are detected regularly in poultry. Highly pathogenic strains have been isolated globally but infrequently reported; outbreaks of the disease in poultry can usually be controlled and eradicated by classical control methods.

The current highly pathogenic avian influenza (HPAI) strain H5N1, however, has caused an unprecedented situation, spreading over three continents, with severe economic and social consequences. Millions of poultry have been killed or died, and many people have lost their livelihoods. Poverty has increased in affected areas in developing countries. Although financial resources have been targeted to human health rather than animal health in the face of a possible human pandemic, the main message of the World Organisation for Animal Health (OIE) and the Food and

Agricultural Organisation (FAO), supported by the World Health Organization (WHO), is that the virus load in the environment and therefore the risk of a pandemic should be diminished by eradicating the virus at its animal source. Vaccination is one of the most important tools that can be used to achieve this goal [1,2].

Initial Strategy: Eradication at the Animal Source of the Disease

To reduce the virus load and circulation in poultry and its spread to unaffected areas and countries, the OIE strategy focuses on the following key actions: early warning, early detection, rapid confirmation of suspected cases, rapid response and rapid and transparent notification. All countries should be able to implement these actions for transboundary animal disease control. Rapid response includes various aspects, such as humane culling of infected animals, containment, movement control and increased biosecurity. Vaccination can be a valuable additional tool in the response, when necessary and appropriate.

Experience gained since the onset of the current avian influenza crisis in 2003 has shown that H5N1 HPAI is difficult to control, especially in countries that cannot rapidly detect and respond to an outbreak. High-quality veterinary services are the basis of animal disease control and eradication, and severe limitations to effective control of HPAI are found in developing countries and those with economies in transition, many of which have either no veterinary services or services that are understaffed and with insufficient financial resources.

Proper legislation and a clear national chain of command are essential for good animal disease control. This is often difficult to achieve in countries with a highly decentralized political structure. A compensation policy of which animal owners are aware is a good incentive for reporting disease. Animal owners who know that they will not be compensated for their losses when their animals are culled will probably choose a financially better option than reporting the disease, like selling diseased animals or eating them. In countries with weak veterinary services, where it is difficult to implement classical control methods, it will also be difficult to implement a good vaccination programme that includes monitoring of vaccinated animals for field virus circulation. Such countries often also do not have good laboratory capacity with adequate personnel and financial resources. As HPAI is a global problem, international solidarity in combating the disease is essential.

OIE Standards and Guidelines on Vaccination Against Highly Pathogenic Avian Influenza

As the international standard-setting body for animal health, the OIE has defined standards on notification, trade aspects and surveillance of listed diseases. The aim of the *Terrestrial Animal Health Code* (referred to hereafter as the *Code*) [3] is to ensure the sanitary safety of international trade in terrestrial animals and their products, by detailing the health measures to be used by the veterinary services of importing and exporting countries. The measures are also meant to avoid the transfer of pathogenic or zoonotic agents without imposing unjustified trade restrictions.

The chapter on avian influenza of the *Code* was updated in 2004 to take into account the latest scientific information on the disease. The new chapter differentiates between low- and highly pathogenic avian influenza, defines HPAI as an infection of poultry and gives trade recommendations on poultry and poultry products, like fresh meat, meat products, eggs, feathers and down. The *Code* also provides guidelines for surveillance of the disease.

Several related chapters and appendices also define the standards applicable to avian influenza, such as the difference between an infected and an uninfected country, zone or compartment; standards for declaring freedom from disease; standards for trade; standards for conducting risk assessments; humane methods for killing animals if stamping-out of infected populations is necessary; methods for disposal of dead animals; biosecurity standards for poultry establishments; and standards for the inactivation of viruses.

A manual that accompanies the *Code* is the *OIE Manual of Diagnostic Tests and Vaccines for Terrestrial Animals* (referred to hereafter as the *Manual*) [4], which outlines a harmonized approach to disease diagnosis by describing internationally agreed laboratory diagnostic techniques. The guidelines in the *Manual* should be followed in order to be able to compare results from different laboratories in different countries, and quality systems should be implemented in laboratories. The *Manual* also gives general guidelines on principles for the quality of veterinary vaccine production and guidelines for the development, production and use of disease-specific vaccines.

During the current H5N1 outbreak, the OIE has received many requests from member countries for guidance in deciding whether to vaccinate and in the design of vaccination programmes. The OIE regarded these questions as relevant and convened an ad hoc group on development of guidelines, which met twice. The outcomes were a general information document on vaccination against avian influenza and guidelines for decision-making, including a checklist of essentials for establishing a vaccination programme.

Assessing The Need for Vaccination

Vaccination against avian influenza can be very valuable in controlling the disease, but it is also logistically demanding and costly. Therefore, it is recommended that a careful assessment be made of the advantages and disadvantages of such a programme and the capacity and capability of the country or region to implement it.

The first aim of vaccination is to induce protective immunity in a flock, and thus increase its resistance to infection, decrease viral shedding and decrease transmission of the virus. To be effective, vaccination should not be used as a 'stand-alone' measure but should always be combined with other control measures, like movement control and increased biosecurity, and should provide for an exit strategy.

Current disease situation

Several steps should be taken before designing a vaccination programme for a particular country or region. First, the disease situation in the country should be analysed, including an assessment of the prevailing epidemiological situation and the logistical requirements for an effective campaign. The epidemiological assessment should focus on the risk for both primary introduction and subsequent secondary spread. All results of surveillance of poultry and wildlife for avian influenza should be included in the risk assessment. The status of neighbouring countries and trading partners should also be taken into account. Local trade, e.g. live-bird markets, is seen as a risk factor for spread of the disease, and pet birds and fighting cocks may also play a role. Countries that are still free from HPAI should be aware of the risk for primary introduction of the virus into poultry populations from these sources. The risk for secondary spread is determined by how well eradication measures are implemented when a first outbreak occurs. If the virus is already present in poultry, it is important to focus on reducing secondary spread to such a level that the virus can be eradicated locally. The capacity to respond to an outbreak with classical control measures is an important factor in deciding whether to vaccinate.

Biosecurity

Poor biosecurity increases the risk for primary introduction on farms, and, in general, the risk for introduction of the virus increases with decreasing biosecurity. Some important biosecurity measures are: keeping poultry indoors or, if not possible, avoiding contact with wild birds or instituting management practices to mitigate the risk for contact; keeping only one species of poultry on the premises; excluding pet birds from premises where commercial poultry are kept; using an all in–all out production system; avoiding installation of ponds, which attract wild birds to the premises; ensuring that feed and drinking-water for poultry are not accessible to wild birds; ensuring that poultry workers do not have access to other birds; erecting a fence around poultry houses; admitting only authorized persons to poultry houses; and ensuring that persons change clothes and boots before entering poultry houses. In countries with many backyard poultry, these biosecurity measures are difficult to implement.

Poultry species

The species of poultry reared is an important factor in decision-making, as little is known about the protective titres after vaccination of species other than chickens and turkeys. It has been documented repeatedly that immunity in ducks and domestic geese wanes more quickly than in chickens, so that these species would require more frequent vaccination [5,6]. Inaccurate vaccination may lead to insufficient immunity and the development of apparently healthy virus carriers. The occurrence of human cases can be a reason for starting a vaccination programme.

For poultry, such as ostriches, that are reared in extensive farming systems in which it is often difficult to mitigate the risk for virus introduction from migratory wild birds, vaccination should be considered a complementary disease control measure [7].

If the risk for primary introduction or secondary spread is considered to be high or if the virus is spreading quickly and the classical response measures cannot be implemented, vaccination can be considered as an alternative.

Implementation of vaccination

Once a decision has been taken to implement vaccination in a country or region on the basis of the above-mentioned factors, a good vaccination plan should be designed.

Vaccine choice

First of all, the vaccine strain should be chosen. A vaccine should always be of high quality, produced according to OIE quality standards and licensed by the national licensing authorities. Vaccines should be selected on the basis of evidence that they significantly reduce virus excretion from vaccinated birds if they are subsequently infected and that the product can prevent virus circulation in the target species.

Before a decision can be made on vaccine strain, the haemagglutinin (H) type of the currently circulating field strain or the virus that is expected to be introduced into the country should be known. The haemagglutinin should be homologous between the field and vaccine strains, as it is considered to be the most immunogenic part of the virus [8]. If only one H type is circulating, a monovalent vaccine can be used, and it is not necessary to use vaccines containing more than one virus strain. Bivalent vaccines containing H5 and H7 strains will protect against both circulating H types. If there is a risk for incursions of avian influenza of either or both subtypes H5 and H7, it is advisable to use a bivalent vaccine. The neuraminidase (N) of the vaccine can be either homologous or heterologous to the circulating virus strain. A heterologous N-type vaccine strain allows detection of circulating field virus in vaccinated flocks by serology.

Vaccine strategy

Various strategies, such as emergency, preventive and routine vaccination, can be applied in different field situations. The term 'emergency vaccination' is used mainly when vaccination is used in epidemic situations to create a buffer zone in the area most at risk. Emergency vaccination is often implemented as ring vaccination in a defined area around an outbreak to prevent the virus from spreading further and to protect the environment of the outbreak. In implementing emergency vaccination, it is essential that infected flocks be culled and other measures, like movement control, disinfection and increased biosecurity, are implemented.

Preventive vaccination can be used when a country or region faces a significant risk for introduction of avian influenza, and the risk assessment shows that other prevention measures will not be efficient and that it will probably not be possible to implement response measures quickly enough to prevent further spread. A strategy in which vaccinated animals can be distinguished from vaccinated and subsequently infected animals (DIVA) should be part of such a vaccination programme.

Routine vaccination can be appropriate in countries and regions where the disease is endemic and where classical control cannot be effectively implemented. The primary goal of vaccination can be to protect the livelihoods of smallholders and to reduce economic losses due to mortality and morbidity, but the final goal should be to reduce spread and eradicate the virus. Generally, in endemic areas, it is difficult to control the disease without vaccination. Nevertheless, classical disease control measures should be used whenever possible, in addition to vaccination. The cost of maintaining an effective vaccination programme is a significant factor. Used properly, routine vaccination can be valuable in reducing mortality and production losses. In the longer term, it could also decrease the prevalence of infection to a level where stamping-out and surveillance could be used and the disease finally eradicated.

All three strategies can be used in a mass or targeted manner. Mass vaccination is applied to all susceptible poultry in a country or part of a country. This option can be chosen when it is unlikely that an outbreak (present or at risk) can be controlled in any other way. With targeted vaccination, only defined categories of birds are vaccinated. When there is insufficient vaccine for mass vaccination immediately available or when insufficient financial or personnel resources are available, categories of poultry to be vaccinated can be chosen on the basis of the risk analysis. A decision might be made to vaccinate only certain species, certain compartments, one or more of sectors 1–4 or only valuable parent flocks. A risk analysis takes into account the biosecurity of holdings, the value of the flocks and the extent of the threat of the infection. The existence of compensation in the case of an outbreak will influence the willingness of poultry owners to notify disease outbreaks and will therefore also affect the decision about instituting targeted vaccination.

Vaccination plan

Each country should have a control strategy and a contingency plan for avian influenza and be prepared to deal with any outbreak. A vaccination plan should be an integral part of the overall contingency plan and should be drawn up in advance to identify the logistical, personnel and financial aspects that will affect the campaign. All persons involved should understand clearly the actions to be taken if an outbreak occurs and how the necessary control measures, such as culling and movement restriction, will be implemented. The chain of command should also be clear. An important but often difficult aspect is the cold chain for vaccine storage and distribution. Currently, none of the available vaccines is thermostable, and all need cold-chain facilities. Each country should have the facilities necessary to maintain the quality of the vaccine according to the instructions of the manufacturer. Arrangements should also be made to ensure that imported vaccines do not remain for a long period at customs at the airport. The number of vaccine doses to be ordered depends on the number of poultry to be vaccinated and on the capacity of the veterinary services to implement the programme. A factor that is often not taken into consideration and which is essential in calculating the number of doses needed and the logistics of a vaccination campaign is that follow-up vaccinations will be necessary to ensure effective immunity. The vaccination schedule, the number of birds, the personnel resources needed to give the vaccine and the required equipment should thus be taken into account to provide for both initial and follow-up vaccinations. All steps in the vaccination plan should be communicated to all stakeholders, including farmers, veterinarians, laboratory personnel, consumers, the public, decision-makers, authorities and donors.

Vaccination monitoring

As vaccination against avian influenza does not always protect fully against infection and transmission of field virus, there is a possibility of virus circulation in a vaccinated population [9]. Therefore, post-vaccination monitoring or a surveillance system to collect data on circulation of field viruses, including analysis of possible antigenic drift, is strongly recommended. Monitoring systems can also help to determine if and when vaccine has been applied and the extent of compliance. Vaccination campaigns can still be carried out if monitoring cannot be implemented, although this is not the preferred situation. The disadvantage is that it will not be known whether virus is still circulating in an area, and it will be difficult to plan and implement an exit strategy. Furthermore, when field viruses are not isolated, mutations will not be detected.

Several factors should be considered in implementing a monitoring system. First, the infrastructure to conduct laboratory tests should be available, including laboratory equipment and reagents, qualified technical personnel and quality control systems. Another prerequisite is sufficient qualified field staff to visit farms and take samples. The samples should preferably be transferred to the laboratory under cold conditions. Telephone, fax, data transfer systems, record-keeping and identification systems should be working properly. Records should be kept of the farms that have been visited and when, their location and the type of holding, the species involved, the dates of vaccination and the batches used. To monitor compliance, serum samples should be taken regularly to determine the level of vaccine-induced antibodies.

The main purpose of monitoring is usually to detect virus circulation in a vaccinated population. This can be done by following the DIVA principle. First, serological tests based on detection of antibodies against the neuraminidase of the heterologous vaccine can be used. For example, when an H5N2 or H5N9 vaccine was used in the current H5N1 outbreak, a serological test for antibodies against N2 or N9 could be used. If specific serological tests against a different N type are not available, sentinel birds that have not been vaccinated against avian influenza and that are properly identified can be placed randomly in the vaccinated population. These birds should be monitored clinically, and serum samples should be taken regularly for serology to detect antibodies against avian influenza. As infection with low-pathogenicity avian influenza can also result in positive serology, each positive test should be followed up carefully. When animals show clinical signs of avian influenza, tracheal and cloacal samples should be tested immediately for the presence of field virus, and all dead birds should be tested for avian influenza. When rapid tests are used in the field as follow up, the results should be confirmed in the laboratory. Only the tests described in the Manual and approved by the OIE should be used.

To detect virus circulation in an area or region, targeted surveillance can be conducted in high-risk places such as live-bird markets. As antigenic drift may occur after implementation of a vaccination strategy if the virus is isolated, avian influenza typing should be carried out in reference laboratories.

Legal framework

Some countries do not have an effective legal framework for implementing control measures against HPAI, and it is not always clear which regulations apply to the control of HPAI. Decision-makers should supervise and support a vaccination campaign and should facilitate implementation of the measures. In poor countries, a first round of vaccination could be financed from public resources, but, in the longer term, a cost-sharing policy should be used, and farmers should be informed well in advance of the costs of vaccination.

Exit strategy

Each vaccination programme should include an exit strategy. Vaccination is an expensive measure and is a logistically demanding exercise for veterinary services. When the virus can be controlled by classical methods, vaccination should be suspended. The epidemiological situation should be monitored carefully before an exit strategy is applied. Although it cannot be known in advance whether a campaign will be successful, an exit strategy should be available. In addition, measures to reduce the risk for new introductions should be designed and implemented.

Acknowledgements

The authors thank the members of the OIE ad hoc group on guidelines for vaccination against avian influenza for their valuable work. The members of the group were: Dr Annemarie Bouma (Netherlands), Dr Hualan Chen (China), Dr Joseph Domenech (FAO), Dr Baltus Erasmus (South Africa), Dr Peter Jones (International Federation on Animal Health), Dr Kouame Kanga (Côte d'Ivoire), Dr Stefano Marangon (Italy) and Dr Thomas Mettenleiter (Germany).

References

1 The OIE avian influenza website : http://www.oie.int/eng/info_ev/en_avianinfluenza.htm.

2 Lubroth J: Control strategies for highly pathogenic avian influenza: a global perspective. Dev Biol (Basel) 2007;130:13-21.

3 OIE: Terrestrial Animal Health Code, 15th Ed, Paris, World Organisation for Animal Health, 2006; http://www.oie.int/eng/normes/mcode/en_sommaire.htm.

4 OIE: Manual of Diagnostic Tests and Vaccines of Terrestrial Animals, 5th Ed, Paris, World Organisation for Animal Health, 2004 http://www.oie.int/eng/normes/mmanual/A_summry.htm.

5 Swayne DE: Principles for vaccine protection in chickens and domestic waterfowl against avian influenza: emphasis on Asian H5N1 high pathogenicity avian influenza. Ann NY Acad Sci 2006;1081:174-181.

6 Philippa JD, Munster VJ, Bolhuis H, Bestebroer TM, Schaftenaar W, Beyer WE, Fouchier RA, Kuiken T, Osterhaus AD: Highly pathogenic avian influenza (H7N7): vaccination of zoo birds and transmission to non-poultry species. Vaccine 2005;23:5743-5750.

7 Sinclair M, Brückner GK, Kotze JJ: Avian influenza in ostriches: epidemiological investigation in Western Cape Province of South Africa. Vet Ital 2006;42:69-76.

8 Veits J, Wiesner D, Fuchs W, Hoffmann B, Granzow H, Starick E, Mundt E, Schirrmeier H, Mebatsion T, Mettenleiter TC, Romer-Oberdorfer A: Newcastle disease virus expressing H5 hemagglutinin gene protects chickens against Newcastle disease and avian influenza. Proc Natl Acad Sci USA 2006; 103:8197-8202.

9 van der Goot JA, Koch G, de Jong MC, van Boven M: Quantification of the effect of vaccination on transmission of avian influenza (H7N7) in chickens. Proc Natl Acad Sci USA 2005;102:18141-18146.

Dr. Christianne Bruschke, World Organisation for Animal Health (OIE), 12, Rue de Prony, 75017 Paris, France
E-mail: c.bruschke@oie.int

Dodet B and the Scientific & Technical Department of the OIE (eds): Vaccination: A Tool for the Control of Avian Influenza. Dev Biol (Basel). Basel, Karger, 2007, vol 130, p 31.

SESSION II

Review of Experiences

Chairperson: *B.M. Seck,* FAO, Mali

Dodet B and the Scientific & Technical Department of the OIE (eds): Vaccination: A Tool for the Control of Avian Influenza. Dev Biol (Basel). Basel, Karger, 2007, vol 130, pp 33-38.

Experiences in Control of Avian Influenza in Europe, the Russian Federation and the Middle East

I.H. Brown[1], *M. Pittman*[2], *V. Irza*[3], *A. Laddomada*[2]

[1] Community Reference Laboratory for Avian Influenza, Veterinary Laboratories Agency, Weybridge, Addlestone, Surrey, United Kingdom

[2] European Commission, Health and Consumer Protection Directorate-General, Brussels, Belgium

[3] Arriah Federal Centre for Animal Health, National Reference Laboratory for Avian Influenza, Yur'evets, Vladimir, Russian Federation

Key words: avian influenza, H5N1, epidemic, control, Europe, Middle East

Summary: An unprecedented global epidemic of highly pathogenic avian influenza virus H5N1 has and continues to present enormous challenges to the international community for control in the animal reservoir. Enhanced biosecurity, good surveillance, both passive and active, supplemented by strong veterinary services, can reduce the risk for incursion and subsequent spread in free countries. Surveillance of mortality and laboratory testing among wild birds are useful early indicators of incursion of the virus into areas in which domestic poultry are not infected. Conventional control methods used widely in Europe and the Middle Eastern region involve stamping-out, zoning, quarantine, movement restrictions, enhanced surveillance and disinfection. Use of preventive vaccination is increasing in the region. In the Russian Federation, all backyard poultry considered to be at high risk for infection have been vaccinated since 2006. Several countries in the Middle East permit the use of vaccine, although rarely as part of a formal statutory programme. In the European Union, conventional approaches for control have proved effective, but both emergency and preventive vaccination could be used. Application of such programmes would have to be preceded by an evaluation of the risks for introduction and spread and might be restricted.

INTRODUCTION

Until recently, the epidemiology of avian influenza appeared to consist of the perpetuation of low-pathogenicity avian influenza viruses of all 16 haemagglutinin subtypes in wild birds, where they caused little or no disease and spread from time to time to poultry. Very occasionally, the introduction of avian influenza viruses of H5 or H7 subtypes into poultry resulted in their mutation to virulent viruses that caused highly pathogenic avian influenza (HPAI). Since the mid-1990s, the epidemiology of HPAI has become considerably more complicated.

The emergence of HPAI viruses of the H5N1 subtype was first recorded in southern China in 1996, and subsequently a number of incidents were reported involving closely related viruses. It was not until July 2003, however, that outbreaks were reported in poultry in the wider region. These events were the start of the unprecedented epidemic of HPAI virus and led to the spread of infection to many countries in South-East Asia. Many approaches were used to control the disease, which at that time was predominantly an infection of poultry. The control strategies ranged from stamping-out, to vaccination plus stamping-out and to vaccination alone. During the subsequent four years, the virus has remained in the wider region, with variable degrees of success in its control [1]. In parts of this region, the virus is now probably endemic.

The virus has evolved substantially since the mid-1990s, and this evolution seems to have coincided with increased interspecies transmission, so that infection has been reported in a number of mammalian species, including humans. Transmission to humans has occurred through direct contact with infected poultry or contaminated poultry products. In addition, other species, such as cats, small mammals and many wild bird species, have been reported to be infected with the virus. The key reservoir species, especially in South-East Asia, appears to be ducks. These can be refractory to the production of clinical signs [2], although studies with certain contemporary strains have shown that the virus is highly lethal for all species of poultry, including ducks. The ability to produce disease and high levels of mortality in ducks is relatively unusual and has not been reported previously for HPAI viruses.

SPREAD, SURVEILLANCE AND CONTROL IN THE EUROPEAN UNION

Subsequent to establishment of the virus in South-East Asia during 2003-2005, a distinct genetic lineage of the virus spilled over into the wild-bird population. During late 2005, the virus spread from northern China to Siberia, Kazahkstan and then subsequently into Eastern Europe, with outbreaks in poultry in Turkey and Romania. Following the first confirmations in Europe, surveillance programmes for both poultry and wild birds were enhanced. Coinciding with bad weather in the Caspian and Black Sea areas and abnormal migratory patterns of aquatic birds during the following winter, the virus was confirmed in 14 Member States of the European Union through surveillance of wild birds in early 2006. Most cases were associated with mortality in wild bird species. Although more than 700 birds were confirmed to have the virus during such surveillance, only five incursions into poultry were reported, of which four were limited to one infected premises each in four Member States (Denmark, France, Germany and Sweden). Circumstantial evidence suggested, however, that the virus spread over long distances without infecting poultry. A fifth outbreak occurred in geese in Hungary and resulted in local spread, with 29 confirmed cases, principally among domestic geese.

The ecology and evolution and the role of wild birds in the spread of the virus are the subject of intense investigation and debate; however, it is clear that wild birds can be infected with these viruses and can suffer disease and ultimately death. Furthermore, the virus has been detected in wild birds in regions where the infection is absent in poultry. Whether the virus can be maintained in such populations independently of exposure to infected poultry is unknown. The viruses that have emerged since the apparent initial introduction of 'Asian lineage' H5N1 viruses into Europe have high genetic diversity, although they remain closely related. Subsequent to its spread to Europe, the virus was also identified in poultry populations in northern and West Africa. It is highly possible that the virus could spread through the movement of infected poultry or contaminated poultry products in the absence of detection in migratory wild bird populations.

The European Union emphasizes preventive measures. As a result, measures to increase biosecurity and set up early detection systems in the commercial poultry sector have proved relatively successful in preventing the incursion and spread of the virus in the poultry population. Examples of such measures include preventing the access of wild birds to surface water and feed intended for poultry and confining birds reared outdoors. Coincident with this approach is a general increase in passive surveillance of both wild birds and poultry in at-risk areas. Furthermore, areas at higher risk for the introduction of H5N1 HPAI viruses are identified and targeted for enhanced surveillance [3,4].

Factors such as outdoor production, proximity to large areas of open water where aquatic birds gather and mix and areas of increased migratory movement potentially increase the frequency of direct or indirect contact between domestic poultry and wild birds, therefore raising the risk for transfer of the virus to poultry. Enhanced surveillance of wild bird populations for H5N1 HPAI can indicate the presence of the virus in a region. Investigations of incidents in wild birds focus primarily on birds with significant disease or mortality, which are sensitive indicators of infection. In order to establish effective surveillance of wild bird populations, effective interaction has been established between epidemiologists, virologists, ornithologists and veterinary authorities. Furthermore, surveillance has been targeted on aquatic hosts with known migratory patterns, population sizes, density and behaviour consistent with a risk for spread of the virus.

Measures for the control of avian influenza within the European Union are laid down in specific legislation: directive 2005/94/EC [5]. The European Union approach to control has been to establish control zones around foci of infection, including after detection in wild bird populations [6]. In infected areas, the movement of live poultry and poultry products, including hatching eggs, is restricted, with a requirement for the dispatch of fresh poultry meat from such zones. In addition, biosecurity and surveillance are enhanced to prevent incursion of the virus into the poultry sector.

Vaccination in the European Union

A Member State may introduce emergency vaccination of poultry or other captive birds as a short-term measure to contain an outbreak when a risk assessment indicates a significant, immediate possibility of virus spread. Such measures must, however, be accompanied by submission of a formal plan to the European Commission for its approval. Similarly, preventive vaccination as a long-term measure is subject to prior approval. Following the incursion of H5N1 HPAI, vaccination was used on a limited scale, equivalent to < 0.1% of the total poultry population.

In northern Italy, bivalent vaccine was administered to laying hens and meat turkeys up to the end of 2006. Two pilot vaccination programmes have been conducted: in one département of France at high risk for introduction, which targeted ducks and geese, and in one in The Netherlands, which involved vaccination of hobby poultry and organic laying hens. In the latter programme, vaccinated birds could be raised outdoors but unvaccinated birds had to be confined at certain periods. Vaccination could be done only in accordance with a 'differentiation of infected from vaccinated animals' strategy. A research-oriented vaccination plan was approved in mid-2006 in Germany, to be conducted in three different poultry production systems and species. Vaccine field efficacy is to be evaluated in laboratory challenge trials, which will be concluded by mid-2008.

Currently, 17 European Union Member States have a policy of preventive vaccination for zoo birds only.

Control in other European Countries and the Russian Federation

Numerous other countries in Europe as a whole experienced incursions of virus, either through wild birds or poultry. The most significant incidents occurred in Romania, predominantly in backyard flocks, and in Turkey, where there were 229 outbreaks, also mainly in the backyard sector. Generally, the strategies used in these countries were consistent with the approaches used in the European Union, i.e. stamping-out without vaccination and movement and quarantine controls. In the Russian Federation in 2005, infection was found predominantly in wild aquatic birds in late summer, but there was some spill-over into backyard flocks, particularly where they came into close contact with wild birds, as is typical in rural communities in the eastern part of the country. At this time, stamping-out was the approved control method, supplemented by movement restrictions, quarantine and disinfection; vaccination was prohibited. Following further incursions of virus in early 2006 and in anticipation of increased spread via migratory birds, surveillance programmes were enhanced, and a Federal programme for targeted vaccination was introduced. The vaccine was given to free-range poultry of several species and to other captive birds in areas perceived to be at high risk of infection due to their proximity to the commercial sector or migratory flyways. A total of 150 million doses were administered between March and June 2006, mainly of a local strain, A/duck/Novosibirsk/02/05. Although there were further cases in the spring and summer of 2006, all were reported in unvaccinated poultry. Further new outbreaks have occurred in the western part of the Russian Federation since February 2007.

Control in the Middle East Region

Since August 2005, several countries of the Middle East region have reported infection, including Afghanistan, India, Iraq, the Islamic Republic of Iran, Israel, Jordan, Kazakhstan, Kuwait, Pakistan, Palestine and Saudi Arabia. In all of these countries except the Islamic Republic of Iran, infection was confined to domestic poultry. Afghanistan and Pakistan experienced outbreaks during 2006 and 2007.

Measures in the region varied among countries, but most followed a stamping-out policy, supported by quarantine, movement restrictions and, in some cases, zoning. Enhancement of surveillance depended on the veterinary infrastructure and resources, varying greatly from country to country. Some surveillance focused on detection of virus, while other systems made greater use of serology. Increasingly, there has been a trend to permitting the use of vaccine, although in some countries a statutory policy may be lacking. Even though the use of vaccine is permitted in several of thes countries, an active vaccination programme has not been applied. Nevertheless, as the virus becomes endemic in some sectors, there may be greater pressure for use of vaccination to control the disease.

Conclusions

Enhanced biosecurity, good passive and active surveillance and strong veterinary services can reduce the risk for incursion and subsequent spread in free countries. Application of a stamping-out policy immediately after detection is critical for effective disease control. Perhaps of greater concern is re-emergence of the virus in a number of countries, raising questions about the mode of spread and the routes of infection, which might vary from region to region. Incursions and apparent virus persistence in the Middle East indicate that the virus might become endemic in some areas, and recent re-emergence in Europe raises fears about the long-term success of maintaining control. With increased spread over wider geographical areas, the use of vaccination is being investigated and used to control infection. A number of issues will, however, affect this approach, including the selection of vaccine strains, the type of vaccine, application of a 'differentiation of infected from vaccinated animals' strategy, appropriate regimes, target populations, duration of immunity and protection, surveillance of immunized populations and thorough epidemiological monitoring of disease status. Vaccination can be considered useful in certain settings to complement other approaches, including enhanced biosecurity.

References

1 Capua I, Alexander DJ: Avian influenza—a moving target. IRV 2006;1:11-18.

2 Sturm-Ramirez KM, Hulse-Post DJ, Govorkova EA, Humberd J, Seiler P, Puthavathana P, Buranathai C, Nguyen TD, Chaisingh A, Long HT, Naipospos TSP, Chen H, Ellis TM, Guan Y, Peiris JSM, Webster RG: Are ducks contributing to the endemicity of highly pathogenic H5N1 influenza virus in Asia? J Virol 2005;79:11269-11279.

3 European Commission: Commission Decision 2006/101/EC of 6 February 2006 on the implementation of survey programmes for avian influenza in poultry and wild birds to be carried out in the Member States in 2006. Official Journal of the European Union 2006;L 46:40.

4 European Commission: European Commission Decision 2007/268/EC of 13 April 2007 on the implementation of surveillance programmes for avian influenza in poultry and wild birds to be carried out in the Member States and amending Decision 2004/450/EC (surveillance guidelines for 2007, published after meeting, but adopted at that time). Official Journal of the European Union 2007;L 115:3.

5 European Commission: Council Directive 2005/94/EC of 20 December 2005 on Community measures for the control of avian influenza and repealing Directive 92/40/EEC. Official Journal of the European Union 2006;L 10:16.

6 European Commission: European Commission Decision 2006/563/EC of 11 August 2006 concerning certain protection measures in relation to highly pathogenic avian influenza of subtypeH5N1 in wild birds in the Community and repealing Decision 2006/115/EC. Official Journal of the European Union 2006;L 222:11.

Dr. Ian Brown, Veterinary Laboratories Agency-Weybridge, Addlestone, Surrey, KT15 3NB, UK
E-mail: i.h.brown@vla.defra.gsi.gov.uk

Dodet B and the Scientific & Technical Department of the OIE (eds): Vaccination: A Tool for the Control of Avian Influenza. Dev Biol (Basel). Basel, Karger, 2007, vol 130, pp 39-43.

Experience in Control of Avian Influenza in Asia

L.D. Sims

Asia Pacific Veterinary Information Services Pty Ltd, Palm Cove, Queensland, Australia

Keywords: avian influenza, HPAI, H5N1, vaccination, control, Asia

Summary: Highly pathogenic H5N1 avian influenza viruses have been circulating in Asia for over ten years, providing considerable experience on which to base appropriate long-term strategies for their control. Experience in Hong Kong SAR demonstrates that existing production and marketing practices should be changed and a range of parallel measures used. It also shows the extent of surveillance required to ensure continuing freedom from infection. Certain high-risk practices should be changed or otherwise overcome in order to control and prevent disease, including intensive rearing of large numbers of poultry in premises without biosecurity commensurate with the level of risk for exposure; complex market chains involving many smallholders selling poultry through large numbers of transporters and middlemen in poorly regulated live poultry markets; and rearing of large numbers of ducks outdoors. These high-risk practices are compounded by weak veterinary services and poor reporting systems. In many parts of Asia, these methods of rearing and marketing are an integral way of life, support the poorest members of the community or cannot be changed quickly without severe socioeconomic consequences. The gains made so far will be ephemeral unless there is a shift from an emergency focus to one of consolidation in which these high-risk practices are identified and sustainable measures implemented to minimize the risks they pose, taking account of the socioeconomic effects of interventions. Vaccination will play a key role, as it currently does in China and Viet Nam.

INTRODUCTION

Highly pathogenic avian influenza (HPAI) viruses of the H5N1 subtype have been circulating in Asia for at least 10 years [1]. They were first identified in 1996, when cases of infection were detected in geese in Guangdong Province in China. This was followed by the detection of infection of poultry and humans by a related reassortant virus in Hong Kong SAR in 1997. Viruses similar to those detected in1996 continued to circulate in mainland China, and, by 2000, reassortant viruses were detected in ducks. In 2001, disease was again detected in terrestrial poultry in live markets in Hong Kong. By this time, infection with various genotypes of H5N1 HPAI was occurring in an arc extending from Viet Nam to Shanghai and beyond, yet disease was reported only in Hong Kong. Further cases of infection were detected in poultry in 2002 and early 2003, and by early 2004 transboundary spread of H5N1 HPAI had been reported in a number of South-East Asian and East Asian countries. Widespread infection preceded the first report of disease in many of these countries. This was not always recognized or acknowledged and led to the implementation of certain inappropriate emergency control measures. In effect, H5N1 HPAI was endemic and widespread in a number of countries, yet the authorities still mounted an emergency response to the disease better suited to places in which infection had just occurred.

Experience from Hong Kong SAR

Experience with H5N1 HPAI in Hong Kong provides a benchmark against which control activities against this infection can be measured. This does not mean that the measures adopted in Hong Kong should or can be copied and transposed to other places, given Hong Kong's small poultry population and small number of farms and the resources available to combat the disease. Nevertheless, this experience demonstrates that different approaches to control can be effective and that there is no 'one size fits all' control strategy; it also provides vital information on the extent of the measures required to ensure freedom from infection in a high-risk area, including changes to marketing and production practices. Most Asian countries do not have the resources or the control over the poultry subsector to make all of these changes. Perhaps the key lesson from Hong Kong's experiences is that, in high-risk places, vaccines have an important role to play in reducing the risk for infection.

In December 1997, when multiple zoonotic cases of infection associated with infected poultry had occurred, the approach adopted in Hong Kong was mass culling, combined with other measures to reduce the likelihood of recurrence. These included segregated production, transport and marketing of domestic waterfowl, a ban on the sale of wild birds on poultry stalls in retail markets, restrictions on farms allowed to supply poultry, introduction of plastic transport cages to replace the wooden ones which were impossible to clean and disinfect properly, mandatory cleaning systems for these cages, and closure of temporary holding farms used to keep poultry numbers to market requirements (so-called 'chicken inns'). This resulted in freedom from infection of terrestrial poultry in commercial farms for 3 years, although some cases of silent infection were detected in domestic geese and ducks imported to the segregated duck and goose market from Guangdong Province between 1999 and 2001.

By 2001, infection with a range of new genotypes had returned to terrestrial poultry in markets. These viruses were eliminated from Hong Kong by depopulation, cleaning and closure of markets, cessation of poultry trade for 1 month and introduction of additional measures, such as monthly rest days on which all retail markets were required to sell all remaining live poultry and thoroughly clean and disinfect their stalls.

Infection on farms in 2002 was eliminated by movement control, culling and ring vaccination, supported by a compulsory enhancement of farm biosecurity enforced through farm licence conditions and prevention of live poultry sales directly to retail outlets from farms. Subsequent outbreaks in 2003 were contained by minimal culling on infected farms coupled with vaccination and subsequent introduction of compulsory vaccination of all commercial poultry (both local and imported). This requirement was fully implemented in late 2003, since when, no new cases of infection have been detected by intensive monitoring in commercial poultry in live markets. This gain occurred despite the persistence of infection in the region, including outbreaks of disease in neighbouring provinces of China from which day-old and market-weight chickens were imported, and the detection of infection in dead free-flying non-domesticated birds in Hong Kong each winter since 2004.

The surveillance system for avian influenza in Hong Kong is perhaps the most comprehensive in the world. It consists of routine virus detection in dead poultry in wholesale and retail markets; tests on sentinel poultry in all immunized flocks of chickens; assessment of all poultry for evidence of vaccine-induced antibody prior to sale; and routine market swabs, which have proven extremely useful for detecting silent infection in markets. Silent infection probably represents incubation of disease rather than subclinical infection and probably occurs as a result of the rapid turnover of chickens in market stalls.

Routine serological testing for differentiation of infected from vaccinated animals (DIVA) was not implemented. Although this was feasible, as the vaccine used contains a heterologous neuraminidase subtype (N2), the use of sentinel poultry was preferred. As all meat chickens in Hong Kong are reared in cages, it was relatively easy to identify and locate unvaccinated sentinel chickens. Unvaccinated animals provide equivalent and more immediate information about the status of the flock at the time of sale. The main reasons for this decision were the complexities of interpreting tests for DIVA, including the potential for cross-reactions with other avian influenza viruses known to be circulating in the region, such as low-pathogenicity H6N1 viruses, and the fact that serological testing for differentiation would only provide historical evidence of infection at the time poultry were due to be sent to live markets, given the lag time between exposure of a flock to virus and seroconversion, which can exceed 17 days. In addition, no formal studies have been conducted on the relative value of DIVA testing for detection of H5N1 HPAI in vaccinated flocks of chickens over alternative methods, such as routine testing of dead birds. Preliminary observations from one small challenge trial conducted in Hong Kong on vaccinated chickens with low or undetectable antibody titres suggest that vaccinated poultry with a poor antibody response are more likely to die than become silent, short-term virus carriers after challenge (T. Ellis, personal communication). This issue warrants further investigation.

Some key observations that have emerged from the outbreaks in Hong Kong have been reinforced in respect of outbreaks elsewhere in Asia. Housing large numbers of poultry in high-risk areas without commensurate high-level biosecurity practices will eventually result in disease, even when biosecurity standards are set. In areas with high poultry density, this will probably lead to the spread of infection to other farms. Uncontrolled trade in poultry in poorly regulated live markets is a high-risk activity. This risk can be miminized if changes are made in the way poultry are reared and marketed, with better traceability and restrictions on entry to markets, and through appropriate use of vaccines.

The detection of subclinically infected ducks in Hong Kong in 2000 and 2001 gave the first indication of the role of domestic ducks in the carriage of H5N1 HPAI viruses. Free-flying birds can also play a role in the spread of H5N1 HPAI, as has been demonstrated by isolation of these viruses from a range of dead birds in Hong Kong. Circumstantial evidence suggests that some infection results from illegal trade in birds destined for religious release, but the precise role of this activity remains to be determined.

Findings Elsewhere in Asia

The measures used in Asia to control avian influenza include stamping-out (usually but not always with some form of compensation), movement management, changes to production and marketing practices, enhancement of farm biosecurity, vaccination, cleaning and disinfection. These are supported by surveillance programmes and communication campaigns. In most countries, combinations of measures have been implemented, and it is difficult to ascribe apparent improvements in the levels of avian and human disease to a specific measure. For example, vaccination was introduced in Viet Nam at the same time as a number of other measures, including market closures and bans on duck breeding.

It became clear in the winter of 2006-2007 that gains made in the control of HPAI can be ephemeral unless additional measures are implemented, such as improved farm biosecurity and changes to production and marketing systems. A number of countries that had previously stamped-out and eliminated infection were reinfected, demonstrating that, although stamping-out can be successful, especially if it is performed when infection is detected early and is not widespread, the gains can be short-lived in places at high risk of infection. Both Japan and the Republic of Korea reported outbreaks of disease in late 2006 or early 2007. The origin of these outbreaks has not been determined; however, circumstantial evidence suggests that both may have resulted from introduction by wild birds, given the timing of the outbreaks, the lack of known connections between most of the infected farms and the strain of virus involved. This situation was similar to that in the same countries in 2003-2004 when wild birds were also suspected, but never proven, to be the source of introduction of viruses. In 2006–2007, poultry farmers in these countries in areas frequented by wild birds were aware of the potential risk of virus incursion, yet cases of disease still occurred on commercial farms. This again demonstrates that measures such as farm biosecurity reduce but do not eliminate the risk for infection.

Among the high-risk production practices in Asia is the rearing of millions of ducks on harvested paddy fields. This activity forms an integral part of traditional farming systems, providing valuable economic and environmental contributions to rural households. Therefore, alternative means need to be found to control infection in these birds, and vaccination is one of the few options available. This is not always easy to implement, particularly for ducks that move from field to field before they are allowed out to graze. Control of HPAI in Asia is also complicated by the complex market chains through which many smallholders sell poultry, involving many traders and middlemen, into poorly regulated live poultry markets where H5N1 viruses can persist.

In other countries, such as Viet Nam, that have been practising vaccination to contain the levels of infection, virus is still circulating and causing occasional outbreaks of disease, particularly in unvaccinated ducks. Neverthless, the number of human cases of infection has fallen dramatically, as has the number of reported cases of disease in poultry. The poultry vaccination programme in Viet Nam was introduced in 2005, when the country had more human cases of disease associated with H5N1 virus infection than any other country. The objective was to reduce the levels of infection. The programme was organized as a blanket campaign covering all high-risk provinces, conducted twice a year. It was accompanied by an enhanced surveillance programme designed to detect infection in unvaccinated ducks and muscovy ducks and serological testing to assess antibody titres. It was not feasible to test all vaccinated flocks, and it became clear that any post-vaccination surveillance programme should be appropriate to the stage of the control programme, as post-vaccination surveillance in the early stages of a control programme in an enzootically infected country will differ from that in a country nearing eradication of the virus.

China has also been using widescale vaccination of poultry for a number of years, in combination with other measures, including stamping-out in the event of reported outbreaks. A number of genetic variants of H5N1 viruses have been detected in China, including those in wild birds in Qinghai in 2005 and in domestic chickens in Shanxi in 2006. The origin of these variant viruses is unknown.

Many challenges remain in controlling H5N1 avian influenza in Asia. The disease will persist in enzootically infected countries as long as high-risk production and marketing systems are not modified. Over time, these practices will be changed through both government and private actions, as has occurred already in Ho Chi Minh City in Viet Nam, where a ban was placed on the sale of live poultry, leading to a shift to sale of chilled carcasses from slaughterhouses. In order to reduce the social and economic costs for poor households, any changes to production and marketing should be implemented gradually and studied to ensure that the most vulnerable parts of society are not disadvantaged.

Acknowledgements

This paper contains information from work conducted by Dr Trevor Ellis, Dr Howard Wong, Dr Kitman Dyrting, Dr Lucy Bissett, Dr William Wong, Dr Mary Chow and the scientific and technical staff at Tai Lung veterinary laboratory in Hong Kong SAR. Invaluable information and support were provided by Dr Hoang Van Nam, Dr Do Huu Dung, Dr Lai Thi Kim Lan, Dr Nick Taylor, Dr Jeff Gilbert, Dr Astrid Tripodi, Dr To Long Thanh, Dr Guo Fusheng and Dr John Weaver. All of these contributions are gratefully acknowledged.

Reference

1 Sims LD, Domenech J, Benigno C, Kahn S, Kamata A, Lubroth J, Martin V, Roeder P: Origin and evolution of highly pathogenic H5N1 avian influenza in Asia. Vet Rec 2005;157:159-164.

Dr. Les D. Sims, Asia Pacific Veterinary Information Services Pty Ltd, PO Box 344 Palm Cove, Qld, 4879 Australia
E-mail: apvis@bigpond.net.au

Dodet B and the Scientific & Technical Department of the OIE (eds): Vaccination: A Tool for the Control of Avian Influenza. Dev Biol (Basel). Basel, Karger, 2007, vol 130, pp 45-52.

Experience in Control of Avian Influenza in Africa

B.M. Seck[1], *C. Squarzoni*[2], *J. Litamoi*[3]

[1] FAO Regional Consultant, Avian Influenza Early Warning and Early Reaction, Regional Animal Health Centre, Bamako, Mali

[2] African Union–InterAfrican Bureau for Animal Resources–Pan African Programme for the Control of Epizootics Regional Coordination, Regional Animal Health Centre, Bamako, Mali

[3] Regional Coordinator, FAO Technical Cooperation Programme 3017, African Union–InterAfrican Bureau for Animal Resources, Nairobi, Kenya

Key words: highly pathogenic avian influenza, H5N1, HPAI control, Africa

Summary: The first outbreak of H5N1 highly pathogenic avian influenza (HPAI) in Africa was confirmed at Kaduna, Nigeria, on 8 February 2006. Within three months, seven other countries on the continent, Burkina Faso, Cameroon, Côte d'Ivoire, Djibouti, Egypt, Niger and Sudan, were infected. More recently Ghana and Togo became infected. The origin of the introduction of the disease to Nigeria and the other infected countries is still unknown, owing to lack of adequate tracing of the movements of poultry and poultry products and lack of reliable epidemiological data from the affected countries.

The preventive measures adopted in countries free from H5N1 HPAI include selective or total bans on the importation of poultry and poultry products from infected countries. All the infected countries have implemented more or less the same internationally recommended disease control measures including quarantine, stamping-out and active surveillance, while poultry vaccination was carried out in Côte d'Ivoire and Egypt. These control measures, adopted and implemented by weak veterinary services, cannot explain the apparent 'epidemiological silence' of H5N1 HPAI in Africa, and further studies are needed to explain the different behaviour of the H5N1 HPAI virus in Africa and Asia.

Introduction

Towards the end of 2004, after the worrisome situation created by the epizootic of H5N1 highly pathogenic avian influenza (HPAI) in South-East Asia, African countries became keenly aware of the risks posed by this disease to poultry and the public health. On the basis of the conclusions of the symposium organized by the African Union–InterAfrican Bureau for Animal Resources (AU–IBAR) and FAO on HPAI prevention and control in Africa (Nairobi, 14-16 September 2005), the seventh conference of ministers responsible for animal resources (Kigali, 31 October-2 November 2005) requested African countries to strengthen their surveillance with regard to avian influenza. Subsequently, the African countries undertook to draft HPAI emergency preparedness plans. Nevertheless, on 8 February 2006, the first outbreak of H5N1 HPAI in Africa was confirmed, in Kaduna State, northern Nigeria. Within 3 months, seven other countries on the continent were infected: Egypt (18 February), Niger (28 February), Cameroon (12 March), Burkina Faso (4 April), Sudan (19 April), Côte d'Ivoire (25 April) and Djibouti (27 May). In 2007, Ghana (14 April) and Togo (6 June) reported HPAI outbreaks.

The origin of HPAI in Nigeria and the other infected countries is still a matter of hypothesis because of the lack of monitoring of poultry farms and the unregulated commercial movement of poultry and poultry products and thus the lack of reliable epidemiological data. Commercial movement of poultry and poultry products is often advanced as the most probable origin of the disease into most African countries; a role of wild birds was suspected only in the outbreak in northern Cameroon.

The explosion of HPAI outbreaks throughout the African continent predicted by many experts did not occur, despite the limited operational and technical capacities of national veterinary services. The situation still remains troubling, however, especially with the confirmation of new human cases in Egypt and the report of the first fatal case in sub-Saharan Africa, in February 2007 in Nigeria.

Preparation for a H5N1 Highly Pathogenic Avian Influenza Crisis in Africa

In Africa, most domestic poultry populations fall into sectors 3 and 4 of the FAO system of classification, and poultry production is characterized by minimal biosecurity. In particular, backyard poultry have possible contact with other domestic or wild birds and are not covered by veterinary care or advice. Other important risks include lack of information about the precise locations of poultry farms and lack of a system for tracing back or forward the movements of poultry and poultry products and inputs by commercial farms. With regard to the interface between domestic and wild birds, few countries have linked veterinary services with bodies such as nongovernmental organizations, working on the ecology of wild birds.

The African region was regarded as the weakest link in global prevention and control of the spread of HPAI outbreaks from South-East Asia in 2005, because of the weakness of its epidemio-surveillance networks and diagnostic laboratory capability, its poor capacity to respond to emergency situations, the lack of studies of the interface between domestic and wild birds and insufficient sensitization of poultry farmers and the general public about the disease and its consequences. In line with the FAO-OIE global strategy for the progressive control of HPAI [1], in January 2006 FAO launched three regional technical cooperation programmes

(TCP/RAF/3016 for western and central Africa, TCP/RAF/3017 for eastern and southern Africa and TCP/RAB/3005 for North Africa) to support national emergency preparedness plans for possible introduction of the disease into the region.

In almost all countries, preparation for an HPAI crisis started with the setting up of national interministerial, multidisciplinary technical committees to coordinate prevention and control. Generally, the committees were responsible for supervising the drafting of an HPAI national emergency plan. Although such planning began during the last quarter of 2005, it was not finished in all countries by 21 February 2006 in several countries: in western and central Africa, plans were finalized in only seven of 17 countries (Burkina Faso, Cameroon, Guinea Bissau, Mali, Niger, Nigeria and Senegal) [2].

Most of the emergency preparedness plans did not start with a preliminary assessment of available resources and therefore did not include precise data on the location and size of poultry populations or commercial poultry flocks and poultry products. The plans therefore lacked realism, coherence and applicability because they were not conceived as action plans, with different scenarios to respond to all possible epidemiological situations. In addition, few countries allocated the necessary financial resources to support foreseeable activities, such as field materials, training of field teams, laboratory reagents for diagnosis, sensitization of professionals and other stakeholders in the poultry sector, shipment of suspected samples to reference laboratories and compensation after stamping-out. With some rare exceptions (e.g. Algeria, Guinea, Morocco, Uganda, Kenya and Senegal), few of the emergency preparedness plans were tested in simulation exercises to identify their weaknesses.

The Highly Pathogenic Avian Influenza H5N1 Crisis in Africa

Dynamics and characteristics of outbreaks

The origin of the first confirmed outbreak of H5N1 HPAI in Nigeria is still the object of hypothesis. Trade in poultry and poultry products (legal and illegal) and other movement of live birds seem to have played a major role in the introduction and spread of the disease in Africa. Indeed, in sub-Saharan Africa, the scattering of outbreaks followed a route similar to trade routes of live poultry, mostly by road transport (from Nigeria to Niger and Burkina Faso; from Burkina Faso to Côte d'Ivoire), with the exception of a case in northern Cameroon in which HPAI virus was isolated from a wild duck. The involvement of wild birds could not be proven, despite extensive searches for H5N1 virus in samples from migratory birds collected in various large resting areas in nine countries (Chad, Egypt, Ethiopia, Kenya, Malawi, Mali, Morocco, Senegal, Tunisia, Uganda, United Republic of Tanzania and Zambia). Apart from a suspicion in northern Cameroon (H5N1 infection confirmed in a wild duck shot at Malapé), transmission of the disease to domestic poultry from wild or migratory birds was not reported in the other infected countries. The strains isolated in Burkina Faso, Côte d'Ivoire, Nigeria and Sudan showed more than 99% homology (G. Cattolli, Padova, personal communication); the samples from the Cameroon outbreaks were not adequate for sequencing.

After a succession of H5N1 HPAI outbreaks between February and May 2006, an inter-epizootic silence was observed, before the resurgence of new cases in Côte d'Ivoire (on 6 November 2006 in imported turkey hens), in Nigeria (in February 2007) and in Egypt (last outbreak on 15 March 2007). The spread and impact of

H5N1 HPAI were greatest in the industrial and semi-industrial sectors in Egypt (more than 30 million dead or culled chickens), Sudan (close to 2 million) and Nigeria (more than 700 000). In the other affected countries, the outbreaks remained localized and affected chickens as well as other domestic birds, such as ducks (Cameroon, Côte d'Ivoire, Niger), guinea-fowls (Burkina Faso) and turkeys (Côte d'Ivoire). Some cases were also confirmed in vultures in Burkina Faso, Cameroon and Côte d'Ivoire.

Control strategies and their results

In disease-free countries, the main preventive measures taken were partial or total bans on importation of poultry and poultry products, the setting up of national coordination crisis units and the drafting or implementation of HPAI emergency preparedness plans. The infected countries implemented urgent measures that were roughly more or less the same, comprising:

- strengthening of social mobilization through communication;
- strengthening of epidemiological surveillance for early detection and early reporting of new cases;
- outbreak management through control measures, including quarantine of infected or suspected zones, culling and destruction of infected or suspected poultry and disinfection of premises and materials;
- management of the socioeconomic impact on poultry owners, including compensation;
- decreasing the susceptibility of target poultry by vaccination, in Egypt and Côte d'Ivoire (and unofficially in certain parts of Nigeria); and
- minimizing risks and improving the detection of human influenza cases of avian origin.

These actions were accompanied in certain countries by:

- improving biosecurity at farms and on live bird markets; and
- updating zoosanitary measures.

The main constraints to implementing the response strategies were the limited capacities of the affected countries in terms of human, technical, financial and material resources; inexperience in managing a zoosanitary crisis of such importance for public health; and, in some cases, problems of coordination between various services, the absence of a direct chain of command in veterinary services or delay in release of funds for compensation.

Information, education and communication

Until the first cases of H5N1 HPAI occurred in Africa, information on the disease was derived from local news media reports and other sources of information from abroad. The spread of factual information on HPAI followed a structured professional approach on clearly defined strategic axes. On the one hand, the perception of the population was of the imminent arrival of a bird disease that could be transmitted to humans. On the other hand, not enough information was provided on the signs of the disease and on elementary hygiene measures to be taken so as to avoid spread of the disease and human infection. The lack of a national crisis communication committee after the first outbreaks in some countries meant that there was no social mobilization for measures such as the suspension of poultry movements, closure of live bird markets, stamping-out procedures and compensation schemes. Extensive public awareness is slowing down, except in a very few countries.

Epidemiological surveillance

In Africa, the weak structural and operational capacities of epidemiological surveillance networks, with ineffective field teams and lack of involvement of private veterinarians and hunters in surveillance networks, added to the weak laboratory diagnostic capacity and problems in submission of samples to reference laboratories, delayed confirmation of the initial outbreaks. Thus, the delays between the first suspected H5N1 HPAI cases and their confirmation were 34 days in Burkina Faso, 29 in Nigeria, 26 in Côte d'Ivoire, 18 in Cameroon, 15 in Niger, 12 in Egypt and 10 in Sudan. In February 2006, the HPAI laboratory diagnostic capacity in sub-Sahara Africa was limited to laboratories in Vom (Nigeria), Niamey (Niger), Bingerville (Côte d'Ivoire), Khartoum (Sudan), Onderstepoort (South Africa) and Dakar (Senegal). These weaknesses impeded implementation of active disease surveillance in the countries where the disease was reported. In most other counties, surveillance is limited to passive surveillance.

Outbreak management

The main disease control measures used have been quarantine, culling, destruction of poultry products and disinfection of infected premises and materials. Implementation of these measures was often limited by imperfect control of poultry and poultry product movements, the non-closure of poultry markets, difficulty in achieving proper border control and, sometimes, selective culling of poultry in infected areas (e.g. sparing commercial farms). In addition, considerable lags occurred between confirmation of disease outbreak and the commencement of stamping-out (45 days in Cameroon and 40 days in Niger).

In Nigeria, in spite of the measures taken, HPAI has continued to spread to most parts of the country (21 of 37 states were infected by 13 February 2007), and one human death was confirmed in February 2007. The constraints to HPAI control in Nigeria include inadequate logistics for disease control in general, inability to control the movement of poultry and poultry products from infected to new areas, flooding of the national diagnostic laboratory with samples thus affecting its capacity for prompt diagnosis, minimal public awareness about HPAI control, long delays in the release of compensation funds and the decentralized nature of the veterinary services, with no adequate coordination between the Federal and state governments.

In Egypt, where 21 of the 27 governorates are infected, similar difficulties are being experienced: state veterinarians have structural and organizational problems, including lack of direct line of command and inadequate coordination at provincial level, and there are insufficient qualified epidemiologists to manage epidemiological surveillance networks, with the consequence that fatal human cases have been used to trace back to contaminated poultry populations. In both Egypt and Nigeria, there is no veterinary supervision of new poultry farms or of imports or exports of poultry and poultry products from sectors 1 and 2, and little attention is paid to following-up poultry in sectors 3 and 4 or providing animal health care.

Management of the socioeconomic impact

In Niger, in the week 28 February to 6 March 2006, just after confirmation of the first case of HPAI in the country, 57% of the poultry markets were closed, 43% of the markets saw their activities falling by 50-90%, and the sale price of poultry dropped by 50–80%. An alarmist communication campaign before the outbreak and the absence of real crisis communication after the outbreak led to large losses for poultry producers and other stakeholders in the poultry industry. A similar phenomenon was observed in other infected countries.

Management of the socioeconomic impacts of HPAI requires arrangements to allow fast and just compensation of poultry farmers, after culling, to encourage early disease reporting and to avoid the temptation to smuggle poultry out of quarantine or suspect zones. The direct and indirect consequences of bans on the import or distribution of poultry and poultry products should also be addressed to ensure the local availability of these products. Although compensation is recognized by all countries, it is impeded by lack of financial resources and is often limited to coverage of direct losses.

Vaccination

In Africa, although all national intervention plans foresee vaccination against HPAI as a component of the overall disease control strategy, only three countries are currently implementing such programmes: Côte d'Ivoire, Egypt and Sudan officially and Nigeria unofficially.

Côte d'Ivoire implemented vaccination against H5N1 HPAI after the first outbreaks in April 2006. In June 2006, FAO supplied 12.1 million doses of inactivated heterologous vaccine H5N9 (Merial). In February 2007, 8 months after receipt of the first doses of vaccine, 4 million doses were distributed and used, mainly in industrial sectors 1 and 2 (especially on grandparent stocks, layer breeders and layers). Vaccination of backyard poultry in the capital city, initially foreseen in the vaccination programme, was dropped owing to lack of resources to support the campaign. Currently, contracts are drawn up with private veterinarians to conduct vaccination in confined farms with fewer than 1000 birds. In this scheme, vaccine is given free of charge but the vaccination fees are covered by FAO. In the industrial sector, the vaccine is sold and vaccination is carried out at the owner's expense.

Egypt imported over 250 million doses of HPAI vaccine (H5N1 and H5N2) from various manufacturers. Vaccination started as early as March 2006 for grandparent stocks and layer breeders. Backyard poultry are vaccinated by Government veterinary services free of charge, while commercial farms pay for the vaccine. Post-vaccination surveillance of flocks, including sentinel birds, is carried out. Pre-slaughter checks of flocks and post-processing testing are done to ensure consumer safety.

In Nigeria, HPAI vaccines of various origins are used without authorization, supervision, coordination or control by the official Federal or state veterinary services [3].

In 2006, with European Commission and the African Development Bank funding, OIE and AU-IBAR set up a 'virtual' bank of HPAI vaccine on stand-by with the manufacturers. This system allows for the supply of vaccine to any African country within 1 week in case of an emergency. Between December 2006 and January 2007, several African countries constituted emergency vaccine stocks from this bank (around 1 million doses for Cameroon, Mali, Mauritania and Senegal and 14 million doses for Egypt). Before its first outbreak, Burkina Faso ordered 2 million doses of inactivated H5N2 vaccine, which were not used around disease foci as planned for in the national contingency plan.

Coverage of risks for human influenza of avian origin

All national emergency or contingency plans have a public health component, including coverage of the risks for HPAI of the human population, by clinical monitoring of persons in infected premises and those who may come into contact with infected birds. Some hospitals have special rooms for quarantining persons with suspected disease. Department of health services and WHO local representatives are working together to manage this component of the strategy.

By 16 March 2007, the human toll of H5N1 influenza of avian origin in Africa was 13 deaths among 24 patients in Egypt, one death in Nigeria and one patient in Djibouti [4].

Biosecurity measures

Across Africa, the inability to implement elementary biosecurity on farms and in live poultry markets results in suboptimal hygiene on non-industrial farms, in markets and on materials used for marketing poultry and poultry products. Live-bird markets, especially along frontiers, appear to have played an important role in the introduction or reintroduction of the disease in Burkina Faso, Côte d'Ivoire and Niger. Implementation of biosecurity measures and 'good poultry farming practices' are the keys for effective prevention of such epizootics.

Updating of zoosanitary legislation

Few countries have revisited their regulations for coverage of compensation expenses after stamping-out operations, for supporting simulation exercises or for enforcing compulsory vaccination in the zones indicated in their national intervention plans.

International and regional cooperation

Since the beginning of the HPAI crisis in Africa, the region has benefited from support from partners. FAO staff and consultants made more than 160 field missions in 2006 to assess the needs of countries and to propose solutions. Within the technical cooperation programmes of the Organization, five regional workshops were organized to train more than 100 senior managers from 24 countries in epidemiology and wild bird sampling and about 50 laboratory assistants in HPAI laboratory diagnostic techniques. Besides providing personal protection equipment kits, autopsy kits, sampling kits and basic emergency laboratory equipment and supplies to support veterinary services in HPAI surveillance and outbreak containment to more than 20 countries, the FAO has also strengthened the diagnostic capacity of certain laboratories and conducted socio-economic studies with its partners (OIE, WHO, AU-IBAR, World Bank, the United States Agency for International Development and the International Livestock Research Institute) [3].

Sub-regional organizations have helped in mobilizing international solidarity by organizing workshops to harmonize intervention plans, to coordinate disease control and to support the establishment of regional animal health centres with the cooperation of FAO, OIE and AU-IBAR.

Conclusion

The HPAI outbreaks in Africa, after those in Asia and then Europe, have been an opportunity to assess the response capacities and sanitary crisis management capacities of African veterinary services, including diagnostic laboratories. The weaknesses of epidemiological surveillance systems and the limitations of intervention tools affected the response time and the efficiency of disease control in the field. In countries where the movement of poultry and poultry products could not be controlled, the disease continued to spread. Some aspects of the epidemiology of H5N1 HPAI in Africa are still unclear, including clinical disease in domestic ducks rather than chickens in Cameroon and Niger, the role of vultures in Burkina Faso and Cameroon and the role of sparrow hawks in Côte d'Ivoire. Other explanations to account for the absence of the epizootic crisis predicted by some experts, such as climatic factors and poultry density, should be studied.

In the short term, it will be necessary to strengthen national epidemiological surveillance networks and consolidate emergency and contingency plans, with clear policy content and clear guidelines for operational procedures, for early detection of disease outbreaks and early, effective responses. A well-focused, and appropriately adapted communication plan is still needed. In the medium term, efforts should be directed to improving the capacity of poultry producers and other stakeholders to adopt biosecurity measures and improve the quality assurance of poultry products.

References

1 FAO & OIE: A Global Strategy for the Progressive Control of Highly Pathogenic Avian Influenza (HPAI). Rome, Food and Agriculture Organization of the United Nations, 2005.

2 United Nations Office of Coordination of Humanitarian Affairs: Annual Report 2006, New York.

3 FAO: Report of the Joint FAO/OIE/AU-IBAR Mission to Nigeria on HPAI, 3-13 October 2006, Rome, Food and Agriculture Organization of the United Nations, 2006.

4 FAO EMPRES-ECTAD: HPAI Situation Update, No. 135, 16 March 2007. Rome, Food and Agriculture Organization of the United Nations, 2007.

Dr. Boubacar M'Baye Seck, Regional Animal Health Centre (CRSA), BP 2954, Bamako, Mali
E-mail: bmseck@gmail.com

Dodet B and the Scientific & Technical Department of the OIE (eds): Vaccination: A Tool for the Control of Avian Influenza. Dev Biol (Basel). Basel, Karger, 2007, vol 130, pp 53-60.

Experience in Control of Avian Influenza in the Americas

C. Villarreal

Mexico–United States Commission for the Prevention of Foot and Mouth Disease and other Foreign Animal Diseases, Animal Health Direction, Mexican National Services for Agrifood Health, Safety and Quality, Ministry of Agriculture, Livestock, Rural Development, Fisheries and Food, Mexico

Key words: highly pathogenic avian influenza, H5N1, H5N2, H7N3, HPAI control, America

Summary: The outbreaks of highly pathogenic avian influenza (HPAI) in Canada in 1966, the USA in 1984 and Mexico in 1994 led to a clear increase in biosecurity measures and improved intensive poultry production systems. In the past 12 years (1994–2006), there have been four outbreaks of HPAI on the American continent: in Mexico in 1994 (H5N2), in Chile in 2002 (H7N3), in the USA in 2004 (H5N2) and in Canada in 2004 (H7N3). In all cases, the control and eradication measures were based on prompt detection, depopulation of infected farms and epidemiological contacts, increased biosecurity measures and control of the movement of live poultry and their products, by-products and infected material. In Mexico, in addition to the aforementioned measures, the use of massive vaccination allowed eradication of HPAI in a relatively short time in two affected areas of high-density commercial poultry.

Introduction

Some of the main poultry meat- and egg-producing countries in the world are found in the Americas. In 2005, the United States, Brazil and Mexico were ranked first, third and fourth producers of chicken meat, respectively, accounting for 49.5% of world production, and were ranked second, fifth and seventh in egg production, respectively, for 16% of world production. Poultry production is therefore important in these countries, and they have become competitive in respect of other countries, like China, India and Japan [1].

Avian influenza is a particularly important poultry disease because of the outbreaks that have occurred in several countries and its zoonotic potential. The avian influenza virus is distributed worldwide, and the 16 strains, classified on the basis of surface haemagglutinins, are found in wild birds, mainly aquatic, representing a risk for viral dissemination through migration. In most cases, the infection is subclinical; however, the H5 and H7 subtypes can mutate into highly pathogenic viruses in domestic birds, with a huge negative impact on poultry meat and egg production and international trade.

Countries in the Americas have had sporadic cases of highly pathogenic avian influenza (HPAI) since the 1960s, which have highlighted the vulnerability of the poultry industry because of lack of effective preventive measures. The outbreaks led to changes in production systems from extensive to intensive, with confined facilities and a significant increase in biosecurity. Governments set up surveillance and rapid alert systems and emergency plans for outbreaks. Some countries have begun to consider use of vaccination for control and eradication of HPAI in their emergency plans. The presence of H5N1 virus in wild birds and poultry in Africa, Asia and Europe has given renewed importance to monitoring, prevention and emergency plans.

Materials and Methods

Official information from the veterinary services of countries in the Americas where there have been HPAI outbreaks in commercial poultry in the past 12 years was analysed in order to compare their control and eradication strategies, taking into account dissemination, the availability of financial resources, risk levels, monitoring capacity and technological and biosecurity levels at affected and susceptible farms.

Results

Sporadic cases of HPAI of the H5 and H7 subtypes have been detected in the Americas. The cases found in Canada in 1966 and in the USA in 1984 highlighted the vulnerability of and risks to the intensive poultry industry, resulting in modification of production systems and a change to confined facilities. In Mexico, with the 1995 outbreak of HPAI, producers adopted strict biosecurity measures once it was found that separation of commercial poultry from wild birds was not adequate and that it was also necessary to reduce other risk factors by strict biosecurity measures, including systematic disinfection of equipment and vehicles, showers and specific clothes for personnel and appointed workers for each production area. The effects of the disease in Mexico marked the beginning a new era for poultry production, which currently has high levels of technological and biosecurity.

In the Americas over the past 12 years, four countries have been affected by HPAI outbreaks: Mexico in December 1994-May 1995, with H5N2 virus; Chile in May-June 2002, with H7N3 virus; the USA in February 2004, with H5N2 virus; and Canada in February-June 2004, with H7N2 virus.

Mexico

In Mexico, the low-pathogenicity influenza H5N2 virus was detected for the first time in March 1994, leading to a situational diagnosis throughout the country. Serological evidence of viral presence, without apparent clinical signs, was found in commercial poultry and backyard bird populations in one-half of the territory. A programme of replacement of positive flocks by negative flocks began, including sanitary rest periods and cleaning and disinfection of facilities. In December 1994, the disease manifested itself clinically as highly pathogenic; the virus had mutated, affecting 2 million layer chickens in Puebla State, a densely populated zone with 25 million layer chickens on 140 farms. Later, in January 1995, a similar virus appeared in broiler and breeder farms in Queretaro State, affecting 20 million chickens out of a total of 400 000 breeders.

The eradication activities included control of the interstate movement of poultry and poultry products, depopulation of affected farms, sanitary rest periods, cleaning and disinfection of facilities, increased biosecurity measures in farms, use of sentinel birds before repopulation and vaccination of all birds in the affected states and at long-cycle layer farms in states where cases had been detected. Between January and December 1995, 383 million doses of vaccine were administered.

HPAI was last isolated in May 1995, 5 months after initiation of the emergency operation. In December 1995, the Government declared Mexico a HPAI-free country. The estimated cost of the emergency programme was US$ 49 million, covering the operation, biosecurity, vaccination and the value of dead and destroyed birds [2]. As there were no funds for compensation, the value of the culled poultry was covered by the affected enterprises.

Once HPAI had been eradicated, a control and eradication campaign for low-pathogenicity virus began, by establishing free farms, replacement of positive flocks by negative flocks, control of the movement of live birds and products, sampling and laboratory diagnosis every 3 months at farms confirmed to be free of avian influenza and twice a year in sentinel birds at farms where vaccine had been used.

Currently, diagnosis is performed at two official reference laboratories and 19 authorized laboratories. The laboratory tests used are mainly haemagglutination inhibition specific for H5, agar gel precipitation, viral isolation and subtyping and amino acid sequencing. Mexico also has a national campaign for surveillance and prevention of high- and low-pathogenicity avian influenza, which is operated jointly by the official sector and the poultry industry. To date, the only subtype detected in poultry in Mexico is H5N2.

Intensive vaccination was continued until 2005, under the direct control of official veterinary emergency services in all states where low-pathogenicity avian influenza had been detected. Since 2006, the official standard for avian influenza has been to allow vaccination in farms in areas where low-pathogenicity avian influenza exists in order to prevent a new viral mutation.

The vaccine used since the origin of the programme has been inactivated, emulsified A/CK/México/CPA/232/94 (H5N2) strain, which has been highly efficient in preventing the disease and achieved its eradication. In laboratory tests and field experiments, vaccinated poultry challenged with field virus did not become ill but could infect other birds for several days, indicating that the vaccine did not prevent infection and viral excretion, even though it was effective in preventing clinical manifestations of the disease.

Since 1998, use of recombinant poxvirus-IA H5 vaccine has been authorized in Mexico, for application to broilers. Eight pharmaceutical companies are authorized to manufacture emulsified vaccine, and one to market recombinant vaccine. The vaccine continues to be efficient against HPAI and is currently used by some countries in Asia against the disease caused by the H5N1 virus. In order to maintain a homologous antigen to the low-pathogenicity virus, which is still found in isolated areas in the country, the pharmaceutical veterinary industry and the Mexican Government in 2006 initiated a project to develop an emulsified vaccine with the new low-pathogenicity virus strain that avoids viral excretion in poultry infected with low-pathogenicity virus and prevents disease due to H5 HPAI viruses.

Chile

A high-pathogenicity influenza virus was detected for the first time on South America in May 2002. Outbreaks caused by a H7N3 virus occurred in two locations in Chile. The first affected an establishment of heavy breeders, with 617 000 birds in 27 sectors, and the second occurred at a farm 4 km from the first one, with 44 thousand turkey breeders distributed in eight sectors. All the birds were culled, in the first case by 1 June and in the second by 10 June. In total, 18 536 birds in the two affected sectors were culled, and all the other sectors were isolated by biosecurity measures.

The control activities were based on three main strategies: early detection and rapid depopulation of infected flocks; increased biosecurity in all farms throughout the country; and prohibition of transportation of live bird, products and contaminated materials. A monitoring programme was implemented, based on cloacal swabs and blood taken in all commercial farms within 10 km of affected farms for diagnosis by agar gel precipitation and virology. The last case was detected in June 2002, and the Government declared Chile an avian influenza-free country in December of that year. The outbreak lasted 2 months, and 5 months were needed for disinfection, sanitary rest periods and use of sentinel birds. The calculated direct cost was US$ 6.2 million, of which US$ 5.6 million were for culling birds and were borne by the industry; US$ 683 000 were spent on campaign activities. The indirect costs for the export and national markets were calculated to be US$ 16.3 million [3].

Canada

An avian influenza virus corresponding to the current criteria for HPAI was detected in 1966 at two extensive turkey production establishments with a common owner in Ontario. Since that time, turkeys have been produced in confined facilities with rigorous biosecurity measures [4].

The last HPAI outbreak in Canada began on 18 February 2004 in the Fraser Valley, British Columbia, at a farm with 16 000 layer hens. A monitoring programme was implemented, based on oropharyngeal and cloacal swabs and blood sample collection at commercial farms within a 5-km radius of the affected farms.

In March, seven additional cases were detected, and the Government decided to cull 275 000 birds in the focal zone. By April, cases were detected on 18 additional farms, and the Government decided to cull all commercial poultry and backyard birds in the control area and to compensate the producers. In July, repopulation of farms on which the infection had been controlled was allowed. The Canadian Food Inspection Agency received 1100 claims for approximately CAN$ 56 million in compensation. On 18 August 2004, the operation was concluded, with 17 million birds culled. The economic impact for the industry was calculated to be CAN$ 400 million. Altogether, 42 commercial facilities and 11 backyard flocks were found to have the HPAI virus. This outbreak resulted in closure of export markets for bird products to 14 countries.

The actions established by the Canadian Food Inspection Agency were based on three principles for control of the disease: rapid detection of infected flocks (surveillance); rapid culling of infected birds, high-risk contact flocks and all flocks within 3 km; and effective control of the movement of contaminated material (birds, faeces and food) and prohibition of the transport of live poultry and its products across the Canada-USA border [4].

USA

In 1984, an outbreak caused by an H5N2 HPAI virus was detected in the USA, affecting commercial poultry production in Pennsylvania and Virginia. On 23 February 2004, broilers in a 6600-bird flock in Gonzales, Texas, tested positive for the H5N2 subtype. The outbreak involved a single farm, and no commercial farms were affected. An epidemiological investigation began in a 16-km radius around the infected farm. The birds produced at the affected farm were sold to live-bird markets in Houston, where two of the five markets tested positive and three were negative. The facilities of all five live-bird markets were depopulated, washed and disinfected. All poultry establishments in the 16-km radius of the index case tested negative to avian influenza [5].

Discussion

As a result of the HPAI outbreaks in the past 12 years in four countries in the Americas, affected commercial establishments keep poultry in confined housing, have improved their technology and instituted various levels of biosecurity. In Mexico in 1994, the biosecurity measures were deficient [2], and the HPAI outbreak forced producers and the Government to implement a strong biosecurity programme, so that currently all poultry farms in Mexico have biosecurity levels ranging from good to excellent, with an official inspection programme.

All four countries studied had emergency plans against avian influenza, and Canada and the USA had compensation funds for producers to support immediate culling. In Chile and Mexico, the costs of culling were borne by private industry. Table 1 summarizes the measures taken in the four countries.

Table 1: Prevention and biosecurity on farms in the Americas during HPAI outbreaks

Country and date of outbreak	Type and numbers of bird	Indoor production	Biosafety level	Existing emergency plan	Compensation for producers
Mexico, December1994-June 1995	Breeders (450 000)	Yes	Bad to regular	Yes	No
	Layers (2 million)				
	Broilers (20 million)				
Chile, May-June 2002	Breeders (462 000)	Yes	Good	Yes	No
	Turkeys (18 535)				
Canada, February-June 2004	Breeders, broilers, layers, turkeys, backyard birds (17 million)	Yes	Good	Yes	Yes
USA, February 2004	Broilers (6600)	Yes	Regular to good	Yes	Yes

The control and eradication activities in the four countries were based on surveillance and situational diagnoses, quarantine of affected farms, increased biosecurity, control of the movement of live birds, products and by-products in affected and risk areas, and culling in affected establishments and their contacts (Table 2). In Canada, culling included birds considered to be dangerous contacts, and in the USA culling included live-bird markets.

Table 2: Control of HPAI in the Americas

Country & date of outbreak	Control & eradication activities	Considerations for vaccination
Mexico December 1994-June 1995. Government declared eradication achieved in December 1995	Situational diagnosis, quarantine, movement control, depopulation, biosecurity, vaccination	Yes. Few farms affected in high-risk area with low biosecurity difficult to diagnose large area non-exporting farms vaccine available interstate movement control
Chile May-June 2002. Government declared eradication achieved in December 2002	Situational diagnosis, quarantine, movement control, depopulation, biosecurity	No. Although vaccination against avian influenza normally protects birds from the most serious consequences of the disease, replication of the virus can occur.
Canada February-June 2004. Government declared eradication achieved in August 2004	Situational diagnosis, quarantine, movement control, depopulation, biosecurity	No. Large number of birds affected antibodies due to vaccination could not be distinguished from antibodies due to natural infection vaccination could take 2-3 weeks, during which time the virus could persist and spread.
USA February 2004	Quarantine, depopulation, biosecurity, situational diagnosis	All poultry establishments within a 16-km radius of the index case were sampled and tested, and, as of 27 February 2004, all the premises tested within that radius were negative for avian influenza.

The only country in which vaccination was used was Mexico. This was based on a number of considerations. The outbreak occurred in areas with closely sited commercial poultry farms, which made it difficult to diagnose and cull birds rapidly before the disease spread. Furthermore, the affected farms produced poultry only for domestic consumption, so that export markets did not have to be closed. Additionally, a vaccine was available that had been developed recently for use in areas affected by low-pathogenicity avian influenza. Use of the vaccine was intensive in both affected and risk areas, covering approximately 55% of the Mexican territory and 70% of the commercial poultry population.

In the outbreaks in Canada, Chile and the USA, vaccination was not considered, for different reasons. In Chile, it was decided that, although vaccination against avian influenza normally protects birds from the most serious consequences of the disease, replication of the virus can occur [3]. In Canada, the argument was that large numbers of birds were affected, and antibodies due to vaccination could not be distinguished from antibodies due to natural infection. Furthermore, vaccination could take 2–3 weeks, during which time the virus could have persisted and spread [6]. In the USA, all poultry establishments within a 16-km radius of the index case were sampled and tested, and, as of 27 February 2004, all the premises tested within that radius were negative for avian influenza [5].

Conclusions

The HPAI virus was eradicated in Mexico in a relatively short time, by the use of vaccination, biosecurity measures and control of the movement of live poultry, products and by-products. Vaccination can therefore be used for the prevention, control and eradication of HPAI. Vaccine against avian influenza prevents disease due to HPAI, does not prevent infection of vaccinated poultry and diminishes viral replication.

Vaccination against avian influenza should therefore be part of an integral control and eradication programme. In the presence of low-pathogenicity avian influenza that could mutate towards HPAI, vaccination should be used when immediate eradication is not possible.

Recommendations

Before using vaccination against avian influenza, various issues particular to each country should be considered, including:

- a situational diagnosis, level of biosecurity at nearby farms, level and reliability of surveillance, diagnostic capacity for clinical signs and in vaccinated birds, efficiency of passive surveillance;
- capacity of emergency services (quarantine, depopulation, clearing and disinfection, use of sentinel birds);
- capacity to control the movement of birds, their products, by-products and contaminated material;
- availability of compensation for producers;
- presence of low-pathogenicity avian influenza virus and risk for mutation; and
- availability of vaccine.

References

1 Unión Nacional de Avicultores: Compendio de Indicadores Económicos del Sector Avícola, México, con datos de la FAO. Mexico City, 2006.

2 Rivera C, Villarreal CH, García GA, Flores H: La Influenza aviar en México, Memorias. Mexico City, Ministry of Agriculture, Livestock and Rural Development, 1995; pp 39-56.

3 Hernán Rojas O, Rubén Moreira Z: Influenza aviar en Chile 2002: Una Sinopsis. Santiago, Servicio Agrícola Ganadero, 2002.

4 Canadian Food Inspection Agency: Canada's Experiences with Avian Influenza (AI). Part II. 2004 Outbreak of AI Fraser Valley BC, Ottawa, Inter-American Institute for Cooperation on Agriculture, 2005.

5 Animal and Plant Health Inspection Service (APHIS): USDA Gov. Online, HPAI, Texas. Washington DC, US Department of Agriculture: www.aphis.usda.gov/lpa/news/2004/02/hpaitexas.

6 Canadian Food Inspection Agency: Canada's Experiences with Avian Influenza (AI). Part I. General Information, 2004 Avian Influenza, BC Fraser Valley, Control Area. Ottawa, Inter-American Institute for Cooperation on Agriculture, 2005.

Dr. Cesar Villarreal, Animal Health Direction, Mexican National Services for Agrifood Health, Safety and Quality/Ministry of Agriculture, Livestock, Rural Development, Fisheries and Food (SENASICA, SAGARPA), Municipio Libre 377, 6A, col.Sta. Cruz Atoyac México City 03310, Mexico
E-mail: coor.tec@senasica.sagarpa.gob.mx and clvillarrealch02@yahoo.com.mx

Dodet B and the Scientific & Technical Department of the OIE (eds): Vaccination: A Tool for the Control of Avian Influenza. Dev Biol (Basel). Basel, Karger, 2007, vol 130, p 61.

SESSION III

Socioeconomic Effects of Vaccination

Chairperson: *J. Domenech,* FAO, Italy

Dodet B and the Scientific & Technical Department of the OIE (eds): Vaccination: A Tool for the Control of Avian Influenza. Dev Biol (Basel). Basel, Karger, 2007, vol 130, pp 63-72.

Economic Issues in Vaccination against Highly Pathogenic Avian Influenza in Developing Countries

A. McLeod[1], *J. Rushton*[1], *A. Riviere-Cinnamond*[1], *B. Brandenburg*[1], *J. Hinrichs*[1], *L. Loth*[2]

1 Livestock Information, Sector Analysis and Policy Branch, Animal Production and Health Division, Food and Agriculture Organization of the United Nations, Rome, Italy

2 Food and Agriculture Organization of the United Nations, HPAI Control Programme, Indonesia

Key words: vaccination, HPAI, cost-effective, developing countries

Summary: We consider the use of vaccination against highly pathogenic avian influenza (HPAI) in three contexts: as part of a stamping-out programme, as a government-led action for disease prevention and as private insurance by farmers. Poultry systems in developing countries cover all four of the poultry sectors defined by FAO and the OIE, each with particular economic aspects that might motivate farmers to take part in vaccination programmes or to initiate and finance them. Outbreaks in flocks of different types have different potential impacts in terms of disease spread and economic effects, which influence the potential benefits of vaccination as a means to prevent or control outbreaks. We use data from three countries to illustrate the costs of vaccination and discuss measures of cost-effectiveness and ways to improve it. We also consider the question of funding sources and their impact on the sustainability of vaccination programmes.

The Context

Vaccination against HPAI can be:

- part of a stamping-out programme whereby instead of culling many flocks (e.g. within a 1- or a 3-km radius of the first infected premises), fewer flocks are culled and ring vaccination is applied in the surrounding area to halt the spread of disease;

- part of a government programme to reduce the number of outbreaks and the level of circulating virus in an endemic country or region, by applying widescale (blanket or mass) vaccination, or, in a country that is free of disease or has almost eradicated it, by targeting populations considered to be at high risk; or
- used by farmers in a private capacity as insurance against disease outbreaks in their flocks.

Regardless of the motive, vaccination is unlikely to succeed if it is the only control measure against HPAI. It should always be supported by other measures, such as biosecurity of individual premises, control of movement and stamping-out of outbreaks that occur.

Most countries, and particularly developing countries badly affected by HPAI, have mixtures of sectors 1-4 production systems defined by FAO and OIE, which feed into different market chains. Economic aspects of each sector affect the desire to take part in or initiate vaccination programmes. The structure of the national poultry sector therefore has implications for the level of national biosecurity and the way in which vaccination is handled.

While biosecurity in farms in sectors 1 and 2, which have large commercial flocks, is usually good, and these farms can afford to invest in measures to mitigate risk, the impact of a disease outbreak in one of their flocks can be very large, travelling fast down long market chains and necessitating culling and compensation for large numbers of birds. Farms in these sectors are also exposed to risk through trade. They are therefore the most likely to carry out vaccination for insurance purposes or, when involved in a government programme, to vaccinate their own flocks regularly on a cost-sharing basis. When such farms are convinced of the value of vaccination for protecting their investment, they continue to vaccinate each batch of birds. The organization of vaccination on a large commercial farm is relatively straightforward and can be done by private veterinarians and farm staff. The government's main responsibility is to ensure that enforceable regulations exist for quality control of vaccine and for monitoring levels of flock protection.

Farms in sectors 3 and 4 are less likely to perform routine vaccination as insurance and are more likely to be supported by public campaigns with a finite life and an exit strategy. Unprotected sector 3 farms represent a risk, in that their flocks are exposed to disease from wild birds and farm visitors and they supply active market chains into cities. Even though a sector 4 farm is exposed to risks from a number of sources, if it is infected the disease will not spread far, and infection might be a greater threat to human health than to poultry health. A predominance of sectors 3 and 4 tends to be associated with weak animal health systems, in which disease is not spotted and rapidly controlled by stamping-out. Within weak delivery systems, it is also difficult to vaccinate large numbers of birds in small flocks. The cost of vaccination supported by public finance can be very high, making sustainable funding and exit strategies a major concern for animal health planners.

Incentives and Disincentives for Vaccination

Perhaps the greatest incentive to vaccinate is the possibility of reducing the scale of culling, disposal and compensation. Depending on the system and the type of bird, the cost of culling, disposal and compensation for a meat bird can range from about US$ 2 to 10 times that amount. When there is a fully developed compensation system, all the cost can be paid from public funds or from an established public–private fund. In contrast, the cost of protecting a bird might be US$ 1 or less or twice as much with a certification system. The costs for layers, parent stock and rare or special breeds will be higher (more vaccine boosters, perhaps the need for a passport), but the cost of vaccination is still much lower than that for culling. Where the risk of outbreaks is high, therefore, vaccination becomes economically attractive. Viet Nam adopted widespread vaccination in 2005 and has since reported a considerable drop in the numbers of birds culled and the costs of culling and compensation. In the first wave of outbreaks [1], approximately 45 million birds died or were culled; following changes to the culling policy and the introduction of vaccination, no more than 4 million birds per wave have died.

Countries, regions or compartments in which export is important and whose importing partners will not accept vaccinated birds (e.g. any premium market that is free of disease) have a disincentive to vaccinate. This was one of the reasons for Thailand's early decision not to use vaccination in Government control campaigns. Given the relatively short life of most poultry and the fact that no country faced with widespread outbreaks has been able to eradicate the disease quickly, however, countries might consider the introduction of vaccination at an early stage, particularly if compartments could be established with vaccination permitted outside exporting compartments.

Apart from purely economic motives, there may be a social incentive to use measures that limit culling. Loss of birds and the delay before restocking are traumatic for all poultry owners, but particularly so for those in sector 3, who may have borrowed to invest in poultry production and have limited recourse to further credit. In poor sector 4 poultry-raising households, the total income from poultry might not be large but represents a ready source of cash. As cash from selling poultry is often directly controlled by women, gender issues might arise with regard to compensation. Agrifood [2] estimated that half of sector 4 poultry farmers in Viet Nam are poor and 3% of their household income comes from poultry.

Widespread culling can cause problems for restocking, particularly with local breeds, and in some areas this might endanger biodiversity, although the extent of the problem has not been fully documented. Widespread culling causes psychological trauma for all those directly involved. In countries of the European Union, veterinarians and farmers have been offered counselling after extensive depopulation. Reports from Egypt [3] and Turkey [4] showed that culling made veterinary staff highly unpopular with farmers, and similar undocumented reactions have been experienced in other countries.

It is difficult to estimate the benefits of vaccination accurately and quantitatively because scientific evidence of the protection levels needed to prevent outbreaks is limited. The financial cost and logistical demands of vaccination are disincentives, particularly if campaigns are expected to continue for several years. This conclusion should, however, be reviewed in two contexts: the cost-effectiveness of vaccination and the costs and logistical challenges of alternatives. Culling, disposal, compensation and movement control are not easy to organize. The next section provides some estimates of costs and cost-effectiveness in developing countries.

Costs and Cost-Effectiveness of Vaccination Campaigns

Each phase of a government-run campaign can be analysed economically. If a programme is viewed as a project with a simple life cycle (plan, implement, evaluate; Fig. 1), economics begins at the planning stage, with the budget and, ideally (although not always in reality), an assessment of the cost-effectiveness of alternative delivery processes and perhaps an analysis of the trade-off decisions faced by stakeholders that might affect their willingness to participate. As the campaign is implemented, data on performance should be collected, so that progress can be monitored in real time. Evaluation during the programme or towards its end, with production, market and epidemiological models combined with actual measurements, shows how the process might be made more efficient or equitable.

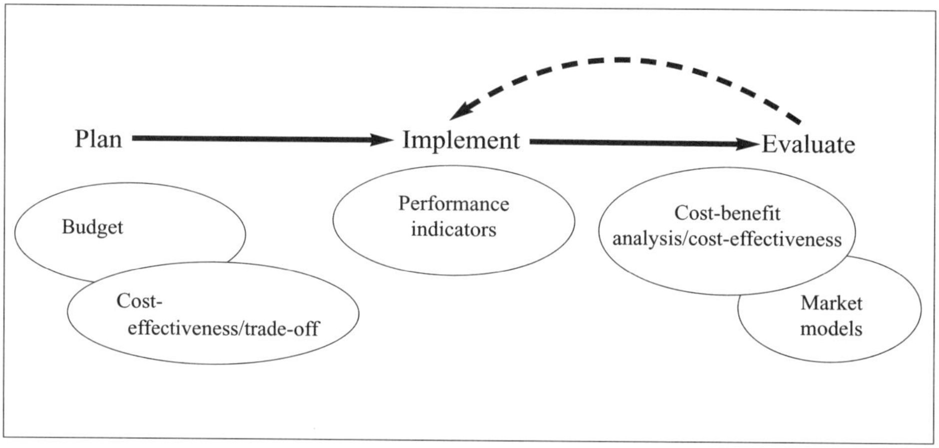

Fig. 1: Disease control project cycle and contribution of economic analysis

Below, we review the budgets and some simple estimates of cost-effectiveness for programmes in three countries where government-led campaigns were combined with independent action by commercial farmers. The countries are Viet Nam, which began vaccination in 2005 when the outbreaks appeared to be uncontrollable, Côte d'Ivoire, where a limited campaign has just begun, and Indonesia, where use of blanket vaccination in selected districts is being considered. The same spreadsheet was used for all estimates, with the input data adjusted by country.

These countries took a decision to vaccinate at different levels of risk for disease. For instance, outbreaks had been occurring for a long time in Viet Nam when the Government decided to vaccinate, whereas the decision was taken in Côte d'Ivoire just after official declaration of an HPAI outbreak. In Indonesia, where HPAI is endemic, the Government is evaluating the possibility of vaccination. The final decision in each of these settings was made under various financial and social pressures, including market demands and political pressure. Our spreadsheet might help to answer a recurrent question that policy-makers ask before reaching a decision: "How much will it cost to implement the policy?" Nonetheless, questions such as the most appropriate moment to change an HPAI containment strategy to include vaccination remain to be resolved.

The spreadsheet was designed and tested jointly by the authors. It includes sections for:

- poultry population (chickens, ducks, others) and percentages of birds to be vaccinated;
- number of vaccinators;
- inputs and costs of vaccination; and
- inputs and costs of government supervision and post-vaccination monitoring;

and output sections showing the costs:

- of vaccination, government staff, post-vaccination monitoring and communication;
- to the public and the private sector; and
- per bird vaccinated.

We consider the estimates to be preliminary, and they will be updated as country strategies change or new data become available.

Viet Nam

Viet Nam has a poultry population of approximately 210 million, although, as in many countries, there is no accurate census for sectors 3 and 4. Nationwide vaccination was initiated in 2005 after outbreaks became uncontrolled in 2004. Vaccination is conducted mainly in Government campaigns, although large commercial farms are increasingly taking responsibility for vaccinating their flocks. Table 1 summarizes the strategy used since late 2005, with three rounds of vaccination during the first year. The strategy was recently modified to provide two rounds, at critical times of the year, with wider coverage. Vaccination is done by private agents under the supervision of Government veterinarians. The agents are trained before they start each round, provide their own transport and receive a fee and a fuel allowance. Investment has been made in a cold chain, training, the salaries of Government staff and equipment for post-vaccination monitoring by polymerase chain reaction. In 2005, investment was also made in mass communication for all aspects of disease control.

Table 1: Vaccination strategy, Viet Nam

	Year 1	Year 2	Year 3
Poultry to be vaccinated per round (%)			
Sectors 1 and 2	100	100	100
Semi-commercial chickens (sector 3)	80	90	100
Ducks (sector 3)	25	70	75
Dual-purpose poultry (sector 4)	60	70	75
Ducks (sector 4)	30	50	60
Vaccination rounds per year	3	2	2
No. of poultry to be vaccinated each year (no. birds x no. rounds)	364.5 million	249 million	255 million
	Sectors 1 and 2	**Sector 3**	**Sector 4**
Vaccinator capacity (birds/day)	1000	700-800	250-300
Investment in cold chain, polymerase chain reaction equipment, vaccination equipment vehicles and staff for supervision and monitoring			
Vaccination by contracted, trained vaccinators providing own transport			

The total cost (Table 2) was estimated to be approximately US$ 21 million in the first year and US$ 17–18 million in subsequent years. The cost of vaccinating a single bird was approximately the same in all sectors: about US$ 0.06 for all associated costs and about US$ 0.04 for vaccine and vaccinator. This cost is the lowest in the three countries analysed. It results partly from the good existing road infrastructure in many parts of Viet Nam and partly from the low cost per dose of vaccine (US$ 0.02–0.03, and US$ 0.04 in the other two countries). Full protection would cost about US$ 0.12 (two doses) for a broiler chicken and US$ 0.18 for a layer (three doses), if it is assumed that each dose delivered is protective. The vaccinator fee per bird in sector 1 is about US$ 0.015 less than in the backyard sector, but the vaccine used in sector 1 is more expensive. About 63–69% of the total cost is for vaccination (including vaccine, vaccinators, their equipment and transport and the cold chain), and the remainder is for support (post-vaccination monitoring, communication and Government staff costs).

If the costs of vaccination in farms in sectors 1 and 2 and the larger farms in sector 3 are borne by the private sector and the costs of vaccination in smaller farms in sector 3 and in all farms in sector 4 as well as the cost of post-vaccination monitoring are borne by the public sector, the latter will pay 82% of the costs.

Table 2: Vaccination cost by sector, year and per bird, Viet Nam

	Sectors 1 and 2	**Sector 3 (semi- commercial)**	**Sectors 3 and 4 (backyard)**
Average cost per year (US$)	2.81 million	4.52 million	11.36 million
Cost/bird for one vaccination round (US$)	0.055-0.061, similar in all sectors		
Proportion of total	**Year 1**	**Year 2**	**Year 3**
For vaccinating birds	69%	63%	66%
Other	31%	37%	34%
Total vaccination cost by year (US$)	20.83 million	16.76 million	18.58 million

Côte d'Ivoire

In Côte d'Ivoire, the vaccination strategy is planned for commercial and semi-commercial flocks, which make up approximately one-third of the total poultry population of 32.5 million. Vaccination was begun recently in order to protect poultry and human populations and to avoid market shocks. Producers are exposed to risks from previously infected neighbouring countries and from unofficial trade of traditional poultry towards Abidjan. After a previous attempt to vaccinate in all four sectors, which resulted in very low coverage of backyard birds, the Government decided to focus on commercial and semi-commercial flocks in a campaign that might last for only 1 year or might continue for longer. The strategy (Table 3) is for 3 years.

The total cost (Table 4) is approximately US$ 2.25 million in the first year and US$ 1.55 and 1.61 million in subsequent years. The cost of vaccinating a bird is about US$ 0.07 in sectors 1–3 and US$ 0.09 in sector 4. The cost of full protection would be US$ 0.14 for a broiler (two doses), US$ 0.21 for a layer and US$ 0.27 for a backyard bird (three doses) if it is assumed that each dose delivered is protective. The low cost is due partly to the fact that little investment was needed in Côte d'Ivoire, as the laboratory was already well equipped and no additional transport was expected to be required. It is also partly due to the fact that in sectors 1–3 private veterinarians and farm staff carry out most of the work. Table 4 shows that a large proportion of the annual cost is for vaccination. On the basis of the same assumptions about private–public cost sharing as above, the share of the public sector is about 53%.

Table 3: Vaccination strategy, Côte d'Ivoire

	Year 1	**Year 2**	**Year 3**
Poultry to be vaccinated per round (%)			
Sectors 1 and 2, commercial poultry	80	80	90
Sector 3, semi-commercial poultry	80	80	90
Sectors 3 (small) and 4 (backyard)	10	10	10
Vaccination rounds per year	3	2	2
No. of poultry to be vaccinated each year (no. birds x no. rounds)	31.8 million	21.2 million	23.3 million
	Sectors 1 and 2	**Sector 3**	**Sectors 3 (small) and 4 (backyard)**
Vaccinator capacity (birds/day)	1000	1000	100
Investment in cold chain, communication tools, vaccination equipment, staff for supervision and monitoring			
Vaccination by contracted, trained vaccinators providing own transport or private veterinarians and farm staff			

Table 4: Vaccination cost by sector, year and per bird, Cote d'Ivoire

	Sectors 1 and 2	**Sector 3 (semi-commercial)**	**Sector 3 and 4 (backyard)**
Average costs per year (US$)	0.07 million	0.07 million	0.09 million
Cost/bird for one vaccination round (US$)	0.13	0.13	0.14
Proportion of total	**Year 1**	**Year 2**	**Year 3**
For vaccinating birds	85%	86%	90%
Other	15%	14%	10%
Total vaccination cost by year (US$)	2.25 million	1.55 million	1.61 million

Indonesia

Indonesia is exploring the possibility of blanket vaccination in farms in sectors 3 and 4, initially only in districts where the risk for disease of both animals and humans is particularly high (e.g. around Jakarta province) and where the veterinary services are strong (e.g. Bali). The estimate shown is for an average district with a population of about 2.6 million birds. Commercial farms are already vaccinating, although the records of vaccine provided and coverage achieved are limited. The strategy shown in Table 5 might not be that which is finally used; it was designed to estimate the highest possible cost of a concentrated vaccination effort. In this strategy, vaccination campaigns will be run four times a year, covering 50% of birds in sectors 1 and 2 and 80% of those in semi-commercial enterprises and backyards.

The large number of campaigns is intended to compensate for the population dynamics of backyard flocks and the fact that protection levels in semi-commercial and backyard flocks might initially be low, particularly if they are immunocompromised by exposure to other diseases.

Table 5: Vaccination strategy in one district in Indonesia

	Year 1	Year 2	Year 3
Poultry to be vaccinated per round (%)			
Sectors 1 and 2	50	50	50
Sector 3 (semi-commercial chickens)	80	80	80
Ducks (sector 3)	80	80	80
Dual-purpose (sector 4)	80	80	80
Ducks (sector 4)	80	80	80
Vaccination rounds per year	4	4	4
No. of poultry to be vaccinated each year (no. birds x no. rounds)	6.43 million	6.43 million	6.43 million
	Sectors 1 and 2	**Sector 3**	**Sector 4**
Vaccinator capacity (birds/day)	1000	500	125
Investment in cold chain, polymerase chain reaction equipment, vaccination equipment, vehicles and staff for supervision and monitoring			
Vaccination by contracted, trained vaccinators providing own transport			

The total cost (Table 6) will be about US$ 0.81 million in the first year and US$ 0.6 million in subsequent years. The cost of vaccinating a bird in sectors 1–3 will be about US$ 0.08 but will double in sector 4, partly because experience suggests that the number of birds vaccinated in a day will be very low. To fully protect a chicken would cost US$ 0.16 for a broiler (two doses), US$ 0.24 for a layer (three doses) and US$ 0.45 for a kampong (indigenous) layer, if it is assumed that each dose delivered is protective. If the costs of vaccine and vaccine delivery in sectors 1 and 2 and larger sector 3 farms are borne by the private sector, while most of the costs of vaccination in smaller sector 3 farms and all sector 4 farms as well as the cost of post-vaccination monitoring are borne by the public sector, the latter will pay 80% of costs. In year 1, approximately 67% of the cost will be for vaccinating birds, while in subsequent years it will be 84%, because in the first year there will be investments in training and equipment.

Table 6: Vaccination cost by sector, year and per bird in one district in Indonesia

	Sectors 1 and 2	Sector 3 (semi-commercial)	Sectors 3 and 4 (backyard)
Average cost per year (US$)	0.25 million	0.09 million	0.34 million
Cost/bird for one vaccination round (US$)	0.08	0.09	0.15
Proportion of total	Year 1	Year 2	Year 3
For vaccinating birds	67%	84%	84%
Other	33%	16%	16%
Total vaccination cost by year (US$)	0.81million	0.62 million	0.62 million

Conclusions

If it is assumed that most farms in sectors 1 and 2 will vaccinate their own flocks, the Government's responsibility and costs for these sectors will be those for quality control and monitoring. Incentives to vaccinate might be linked to compensation schemes: if there is no compensation, the incentive to vaccinate as insurance will be high; exoneration of a farm with a vaccination certificate from culling of healthy birds is also an incentive to vaccinate. Sustainability is not an issue in these sectors, which will continue to vaccinate each batch of birds against Newcastle disease and Gumboro disease.

If HPAI control is considered to be a global public good, there is an argument for subsidizing preventive vaccination at farms in sector 3. Of all the elements of a control strategy, however, vaccination is that which farmers are most inclined to finance, as it can have private benefits. The cost can be subsidized if the government pays for monitoring and surveillance. Sometimes, the cost of the vaccine is also subsidized, as in Côte d'Ivoire. The incentive to vaccinate broilers is minimal unless HPAI vaccine is combined with vaccine against Newcastle disease. Small, unregulated hatcheries might represent a strong risk of virus spread, and they might be good candidates for vaccination of day-old chicks. Trovac vaccine is, however, very expensive and might justify a subsidy. Alternatively, private benefit might ensue if vaccinated day-old chicks are certified and then sold at a higher price.

A decision to vaccinate on farms in sector 4 should be based on a local risk assessment. This sector is highly variable, and farms should be categorized into 'high risk' and 'low risk' groups. Vaccination in sector 4 is most urgent where poultry and people are dense. In sparse populations, the virus may die out in the absence of strong control measures; vaccine might be used to create barriers to spread and hasten dying out. Cost-effectiveness includes not only reduced cost but also increasing coverage, and this might be difficult to achieve for the reasons described by others in this publication. We must assume that farms in sector 4 will not pay for routine HPAI vaccination. If vaccine is made available and delivered by animal health workers, a charge will be made.

Comparison of the costs per bird in different production systems must take into account different lifespans. For example, broilers have a lifespan of 45-60 days, whereas layer hens often live for at least 18 months. Therefore, although the vaccination cost per broiler was found to be lower than that for a layer, the cost per hen–day protected will be significantly lower for layers than for broilers. It will be important to add such concepts into future models for assessing the cost-effectiveness of vaccination campaigns.

We have not undertaken cost-benefit analysis or estimated benefits, as this would take up as much space again. We used two simple cost-effectiveness measures: the cost per dose delivered and the cost per bird protected. The ideal denominator depends on the objectives of the programme. An interesting measure would be the cost per bird at risk, but this would require better data about poultry populations and epidemiological risk estimates than were available at the time of writing. In countries where farms in sectors 3 and 4 predominate, the transaction costs are high because there are many individual units to be served. This might be a good reason for targeting vaccination to areas at particular risk, either geographically (because of trade) or at one end of the value chain, such as hatcheries. Important factors in cost-effectiveness include the control entity (The protection level might be affected by the producer's perception of risk.), allocation of costs (The cost of vaccine can be subsidized easily, but delivery of vaccine administered by a farmer is more difficult to subsidize.) and the entity that delivers (It is often cheaper to contract out.).

The costs of preventive vaccination are easier to estimate than those for stamping-out, which presuppose knowledge about the risk of an outbreak. Data on poultry populations are, however, usually poor, in particular for farms in sector 4. If census data are not available, populations must be estimated by proxies. Planning for resources must include sources of funds and a reliable source of vaccine.

Vaccination is only one part of a control strategy and will always be used in combination with other measures. Important work remains to be done in assisting affected and at-risk countries to review the economic and social trade-offs in considering use of vaccination and other control measures in a comprehensive programme.

References

1 Tuan NA: Presentation made at a workshop on 'Future of poultry farmers in Vietnam after HPAI', 8-9 March 2007, Hanoi. Rome, Food and Agriculture Organization of the United Nations, 2007.

2 Agrifood: The Economic Impact of Highly Pathogenic Avian Influenza-related Biosecurity Policies on the Vietnamese Poultry Sector. Rome, Food and Agriculture Organization of the United Nations, 2007.

3 Ghonem M: Rapid Assessment of Highly Pathogenic Avian Influenza Procedures for Reimbursement of Backyard and Industrial Poultry Producers after the HPAI Outbreak: Smallholder and Backyard Producers, Egypt. Rome, Food and Agriculture Organization of the United Nations, 2006.

4 Geerlings E: Rapid Assessment of HPAI Socio-economic Impacts in Turkey. Rome, Food and Agriculture Organization of the United Nations, 2006.

Dr. Anni McLeod, Livestock Information, Sector Analysis and Policy Branch, Animal Production and Health Division, Food and Agriculture Organization of the United Nations, Rome, Italy
E-mail: anni.mcleod@fao.org

Dodet B and the Scientific & Technical Department of the OIE (eds): Vaccination: A Tool for the Control of Avian Influenza. Dev Biol (Basel). Basel, Karger, 2007, vol 130, pp 73-82.

Challenges and Constraints to Vaccination in Developing Countries

R.G. Alders[1], B. Bagnol[1,2], M.P. Young[1], C. Ahlers[3], E. Brum[4], J. Rushton[5]

1 International Rural Poultry Centre, Kyeema Foundation, Australia

2 Department of Anthropology, University of the Witwatersrand, Johannesburg, South Africa

3 Food and Agricultural Organization of the United Nations, Regional Office for Asia and the Pacific, Bangkok, Thailand

4 Cummings School of Veterinary Medicine, Tufts University, North Grafton, Massachusetts, USA

5 Food and Agriculture Organization of the United Nations, Rome, Italy

Key words: HPAI, poultry, vaccination, vaccination failure

Summary: The challenges and constraints to vaccinating poultry in areas where adequate infrastructure and human resources are lacking are addressed in both a technical and a socioeconomic framework. The key issues discussed are: (1) selection of an appropriate vaccine and vaccination technique, including the advantages and disadvantages of a combined vaccine against highly pathogenic avian influenza (HPAI) and Newcastle disease and addressing the differences between endemic disease and emergency disease control; (2) vaccine conservation and distribution; (3) evaluation of the flocks to be vaccinated in terms of their disease status, immunocompetence and production systems; (4) design of effective information, education and communication materials and methods with and for veterinary and extension staff as well as commercial and smallholder producers and community vaccinators in rural areas; (5) evaluation and monitoring systems for technical and socioeconomic factors that affect vaccination; (6) support and coordination of and by relevant public and private agencies; (7) the role of simultaneous implementation of other control activities in addition to vaccination; (8) the importance of assessing the costs and cost-effectiveness of various approaches to the control of HPAI, including the prevention of other endemic killer diseases and options for cost-sharing; (9) evaluation of the incentives for poultry-holders, vaccinators and vaccine producers to contribute to and participate in effective vaccination campaigns; and (10) policy development and the organizational framework for short- and long-term implementation and communication to decision-makers.

Introduction

Vaccination is an important component of commercial flock management strategies in many countries, as it is the most cost-effective means of preventing and controlling the spread of economically important diseases such as Marek's disease, Newcastle disease and infectious bursal disease [1]. Vaccination of village poultry in rural areas against killer diseases such as Newcastle disease has become an increasingly viable option with the development of thermotolerant vaccines [2]. Vaccination can support programmes for eradicating diseases such as highly pathogenic avian influenza (HPAI) when effectively implemented in conjunction with other control methods such as quarantine and movement control, culling, improved producer and trader knowledge; improved sanitation and husbandry; improved biosecurity (both bioexclusion and biocontainment) and improved food safety [3]. It is important to combine vaccination with other control methods because the vaccines currently available prevent clinical disease but do not prevent infection. In the case of vaccination against HPAI, successfully vaccinated birds challenged with virulent virus become infected but the bird's immune response significantly reduces the amount of virus shed into the environment [3].

Where adequate infrastructure and human resources are lacking, effective vaccination can be difficult to implement [4,5], as can other disease control measures (Table 1). The issues addressed below should be assessed before and during implementation of poultry vaccination programmes, irrespective of the location in which the programme is to be implemented. The local context will, however, influence the approaches used to ensure optimal results.

Table 1: National factors that can influence the efficiency with which HPAI can be controlled

Criterion	Countries in which HPAI was quickly controlled	Countries in which HPAI control was difficult
Percentage of households raising poultry	Low. Most poultry produced on large commercial farms	High. Many households raise small poultry flocks; commercial farms also present
Farmer–poultry health service links	Strong	Poor
Farmers' perceptions of disease	Aware of the role of infectious agents	Traditional. Disease often thought to be caused by supernatural phenomena
Literacy rate	High	Low
Annual poultry mortality	Low	High
Poultry production quality assurance	Strong	Weak

Selection of Appropriate Vaccine and Vaccination Technique

The ideal HPAI vaccine does not yet exist, and it is important to assess the various options in terms of purity, safety, potency, subtype, thermotolerance, ease of use, labels and instruction sheets in local languages, availability, registration status and the ability of the vaccine to provoke an immune response that can be differentiated from that generated in response to infection with field strains. An ability to conduct quality assurance on vaccines is advantageous and increases national capacity to evaluate imported and locally produced vaccine and to test the potency of poorly conserved vaccine [6].

The technique used to vaccinate birds greatly influences both the cost and the effectiveness of the vaccination programme. It is essential that a robust quality assurance programme is in operation to support vaccination. The cost of vaccine represents a very small part of the overall cost of vaccinating birds. Prophylactic HPAI vaccination is rarely used, and its use should be considered only when there is a high risk of incursion by a known subtype. Emergency vaccination in the face of an outbreak has been shown experimentally to reduce the reproduction ratio to < 1 within 1 week of vaccination [3], and anecdotal evidence from Viet Nam suggests that a similar effect is seen in the field. In terms of slowing the spread of HPAI, emergency vaccination is a useful option when stamping-out alone cannot solve the problem. When the knowledge of poultry producers about disease and immune processes is minimal, however, vaccinating in the face of an outbreak can result in significant resistance from producers if birds that were already incubating the disease are vaccinated and subsequently die.

Most HPAI vaccines are inactivated and must therefore be administered by injection. This presents many challenges. Re-use of needles between birds can lead to transmission of both HPAI and other infectious agents, such as that of Newcastle disease and the reticuloendotheliosis virus. Care must be taken to reduce the risk for needle-stick injury to the vaccinator or bird handler. The oil emulsion in inactivated vaccines can provoke a serious inflammatory reaction in people accidentally injected with vaccine. Vaccinators should be trained to reduce the risk for transmission of blood-borne pathogens through needle-stick injury, and they must be given an appropriate means of needle disposal.

There is no easy way to vaccinate extensively raised poultry. Village flocks are multi-aged, generally cared for by women and children (who are not always effectively targeted by awareness campaigns), frequently consist of different species raised in the same household and can be difficult to catch even when night housing is available. Vaccinating birds from different households in a central location might be easier for vaccinators but increases the risk for spread of disease among flocks. If vaccination is done on a house-to-house basis, the vaccinators must be well trained and equipped to minimize the risk for mechanical transmission of diseases among households. Well-trained male and female community vaccinators have an important role to play when the disease is endemic, as they are the most cost-effective means of administering vaccine on a regular basis. Community vaccinators are, however, often reluctant to vaccinate small village birds and birds under 2 months of age for fear of killing them by mechanical trauma. Therefore, specialists within the group of community vaccinators should be trained to vaccinate small birds. As birds under 2 months of age make up an average of 50% of a village chicken flock, failure to vaccinate them greatly reduces vaccination coverage and thus jeopardizes the entire exercise.

Where Newcastle disease is endemic, control of this disease will facilitate early detection of HPAI. Use of a combined injectable vaccine against HPAI and Newcastle disease is being studied for areas where both diseases are endemic. Better results would probably be achieved with use of an inactivated HPAI vaccine and a live Newcastle disease vaccine given in eye drops or drinking-water, and use of live

Newcastle disease vaccine would increase protection in young animals with maternal antibodies and facilitate horizontal spread of vaccine virus to birds that have escaped vaccination by injection. In rural areas, the best results have been attained by administering live thermotolerant Newcastle disease vaccine every 4 months [2].

Vaccine Conservation and Distribution

The cost of vaccine represents a relatively small proportion of the overall cost of vaccination. The costs associated with training and mobilizing field staff and with vaccine distribution add significantly to the cost of vaccination, especially in remote areas where cold chains are not reliable. It is therefore essential that vaccine dispatched to the field remains capable of stimulating an adequate immune response until it is administered to birds. Where cold chains are lacking or unreliable, it is advisable to conduct vaccination during campaigns, so that an appropriate distribution system can be mounted for the duration of the campaign in a particular area. Potential cold-chain inadequacies can be identified from data loggers and maximum-minimum thermometers before a campaign [7]. Information about the status of the cold chain and the thermotolerance of the vaccine to be used must be provided to teams in the field to enable them to work with confidence.

Where vaccination is to be a long-term activity, public–private partnerships should be explored to reduce the burden on government services while maintaining adequate quality control.

Poultry Flock Profile

Flock characteristics must be determined during planning. Flock disease status, immunocompetency and production systems must all be identified in order to confirm that vaccination coverage capable of protecting the flock and preventing the spread of virulent virus can be achieved.

Birds' immune systems play a critical role in defending them against pathogens. The system comprises various cells and soluble factors that together produce a protective immune response. Immune cells develop in primary lymphoid organs (the thymus and bursa of Fabricius), before populating the secondary lymphoid organs (the spleen, bone marrow, Harderian gland and conjunctival-, bronchial- and gut-associated lymphoid tissue), the principal sites of antigen-induced immune responses. Damage to any part of the immune system leads to increased susceptibility to infectious disease and to an impaired response to vaccine or vaccine failure. Immunosuppressive effects have been ascribed to malnutrition, parasitism and stress, as well as various viral diseases and agents, including infectious bursal disease (Gumboro disease in chickens), inclusion body hepatitis in chickens and turkeys, Angara disease (infectious hydropericardium in chickens), haemorrhagic enteritis in turkeys, chicken infectious anaemia, runting syndrome in geese (a circovirus infection), aflatoxicosis, ochratoxicosis, Marek's disease and reticuloendotheliosis. When primary lymphoid organs are targeted, the impact on the immune system is irreversible, causing lifelong immunosuppression. Diseases such as infectious bursal disease have had a major impact on the poultry industry and remain inadequately controlled in many developing countries [8].

The poultry production system involved must be described in terms of age profile (single or multi-age flocks), breeds, species, production cycles, circulating diseases and current animal health practices to enable appropriate tailoring of vaccination.

Information, Education and Communication

Effective information, education and communication are essential to ensure that vaccination and wide HPAI prevention and control are coordinated and effective [9]. Communication packages must be prepared for a wide range of stakeholders, from senior government and international decision-makers to male and female poultry owners, so that each can obtain the knowledge necessary to make timely, sound decisions that will facilitate vaccination activities. The material should be tailored for the group concerned while retaining consistency of information. When new information is to be prepared, adequate time and finances must be given to enable research, preparation, pre-testing, production and monitoring. The design and monitoring of information, education and communication activities should be collaborative, with participatory methods to promote genuine dialogue, and should be seen as a dynamic process of improvement.

Special consideration must be given to the role of information, education and communication in areas where poultry producers have had little access to formal education, especially when emergency vaccination is to be conducted. To minimize confusion, the translation of technical terms into local languages requires special attention. For example, in many rural areas, vaccination is loosely translated as 'injection'; however, various products can be injected, including vaccines, antibiotics and vitamins. When birds injected with an antibiotic subsequently die from disease, smallholder producers frequently believe that the 'injection' failed to protect their birds or, worse still, that the 'injection' was responsible for the bird's death.

Key information must be given to producers before or at the time of vaccination. One message is that protective immunity takes 7-10 days to develop, so that birds are not protected immediately after vaccination. Secondly, vaccines protect against specific diseases and not against 'all risks'. Thirdly, apparently healthy birds can be incubating disease. Fourthly, not all birds respond adequately to vaccination, so that the protection of all vaccinated birds cannot be guaranteed. Lastly, the vaccine will not harm birds, but mechanical trauma due to injection can engender a risk for small birds and/or poorly trained vaccinators. A vaccination programme therefore requires awareness-raising activities before a campaign is begun, in order to explain the benefits of the vaccine and the risks. These exercises will probably have to be repeated before each campaign. The delivery of the messages could be incorporated into school curricula, especially in areas where information is known to be transmitted by schoolchildren to their parents [10].

Timely, Efficient Monitoring and Evaluation

Monitoring and evaluation are an integral part of vaccination and are especially important in the case of HPAI, as the circulating field strain must be monitored continuously. Vaccine quality assurance confirms that vaccines are safe and potent, that no extraneous agents are present and that inactivated vaccine is correctly inactivated. Ideally, monitoring and evaluation are built into training programmes, so that the persons involved will monitor and evaluate their own activities without waiting for feedback from their supervisors.

Disease surveillance of poultry, wild birds and rare captive birds is part of monitoring and evaluation. Vaccination failure in commercial poultry flocks is a problem in many countries, and failure to perform sero-monitoring after vaccination has delayed the detection of HPAI in flocks in which high mortality was initially attributed to Newcastle disease, even when the flocks had been vaccinated against this disease. To improve vaccination and to gain the confidence of producers, all vaccination failures must be investigated (Table 2). Inadvertent deaths of birds after vaccination due to mechanical injury or other adverse reactions should be recorded and monitored.

Table 2: Factors that can contribute to vaccination failure in poultry

Reason for vaccination failure	**Potential causes**
Vaccinated animals not immunocompetent	Presence of maternal antibodies Prior or current infection with immuno-suppressive agents, such as infectious bursal disease, parasites Birds already incubating disease Malnutrition
Vaccine not effective in vaccinated species	Biological variation
Vaccine not effective	Poor quality vaccine Vaccine past expiry date Poor vaccine conservation Field strain different from that in vaccine
Ineffective vaccination	Wrong dosage Not all birds vaccinated Failure to administer entire dose No revaccination or revaccination interval too long

The socioeconomic indicators to be monitored include perceptions in the community (e.g. of male and female community leaders and vaccinators) and behaviour, impact and cost-efficiency. More data on the effectiveness of vaccine delivery and vaccine efficacy in the field are required in order to make accurate estimates of cost-effectiveness and to guide policies and projects in vaccination campaign management. Monitoring and evaluation are therefore essential for any campaign, and the results should be used to modify and improve future campaigns and existing distribution systems. Thus, the benefits of a robust monitoring and evaluation programme extend from the local to the international level.

Ownership, Coordination, Policy and Organizational Framework

Timely, effective administration of vaccines requires effective coordination in a facilitating policy environment, with sharing of responsibility by all stakeholders, including poultry producers (male and female), vaccinators (public and private), national government agencies, international agencies and vaccine manufacturers. It requires a common vision and communication channels for open and timely sharing of information, all of which are built on trust in and a commitment to implementation of a successful vaccination programme.

Policy and organization frameworks are required to enable public-private collaboration in the areas of vaccine testing and approval, vaccine monitoring, vaccine distribution and administration and training. Short-, medium- and long-term strategies are required that include an exit strategy.

Cost and Cost-Effectiveness Analyses

Effective vaccination (preparation, implementation and monitoring) requires funding, and it is critical that the costs be determined in advance to confirm that adequate funds are available. Vaccination should not be started if adequate funding cannot be guaranteed. Cost-sharing options that include producer contributions should be studied and implemented wherever possible. Financial contributions from producers will contribute to the delivery of quality services.

Vaccination is a complex activity, and financing of vaccine and its delivery must be carefully planned. Some aspects of distribution are best run by the private sector. A vaccination programme should also address the motivations of the vaccinators and, if necessary, provide additional incentives for delivery. The public sector clearly has a role to play in surveillance, to ensure that the vaccine is delivered in a good state and is efficacious. Information on the costs and cost structure of vaccination campaigns for HPAI is scarce. Models available [11] for estimating anticipated costs should be supplemented with data from monitoring and evaluation to determine how well the estimates match with reality. Costs should be combined with epidemiological information to make true assessments of cost-effectiveness. The obvious measure is the cost of delivering a vaccine to a bird, but the most appropriate would be the cost per bird protected (i.e. seroconverted) or the cost per bird-day protected in a population at risk. The former measure requires information from vaccination surveillance, and the latter requires information on the epidemiology of the disease in a country.

Applied Research Requirements

To improve the cost-efficiency of vaccination, applied research is needed to enable field workers to proceed with confidence and efficiency. Research areas include: individual producer factors (understanding poultry production and health, motivations for improving poultry health); cultural issues (gender roles, cultural role of poultry, cultural responses to poultry diseases and control options); socioeconomic and biological factors (flock dynamics, poultry production systems, species differences in response to vaccination, market forces and marketing practices, access to effective information, education and communication by groups such as female poultry producers, cold chain); technological factors (vaccine thermotolerance, novel vaccine technology); and epidemiological factors (appropriate vaccine coverage, transmission chains in susceptible populations and various production systems, timing of campaigns).

Discussion and Conclusions

Mounting and maintaining an effective vaccination campaign against HPAI is complex and challenging. A comprehensive programme can be conceptualized as a holarchy, or nested hierarchy, of integrated activities (Fig. 1), which depicts both the interrelatedness (i.e. dependence) of the various factors in a vaccination programme and the relation of each component to each other. In designing a vaccination programme, it becomes clear that focusing on cold storage at the local level is fruitless unless cold storage is first addressed from the point of production to the point of local storage (hence the cold 'chain' concept). A holarchy also allows for simultaneous consideration of internal factors such as gender issues, cultural beliefs and personal motivation with external factors such as the cold chain and training. Addressing both external and internal factors results in a comprehensive, integral approach to the challenge of successfully vaccinating poultry in developing countries.

Countries that are currently free of HPAI would be advised to improve their ability to prevent or detect and control HPAI quickly and thus minimize the need for vaccination. Proactive prevention and control measures include reducing the overall level of poultry mortality in all sectors by implementation of cost-efficient bio-exclusion and biocontainment measures, including effective vaccination against other killer diseases; active and passive surveillance for HPAI and other killer diseases; improving links between veterinary services and poultry producers; improving access to information and education to enhance understanding of hygiene, food safety, disease transmission and quality poultry production by producers, traders and technical staff; conducting risk assessments across all sectors to identify potential risks and how they might be mitigated; and formulating and testing contingency plans in regular simulation exercises.

The current HPAI epidemic has served to highlight the neglect of veterinary services and small-scale poultry producers, who are mostly women, over the past two decades. There is now an unprecedented opportunity, through HPAI prevention and control, to improve the quality of livestock vaccination and health and production in general. These gains will greatly reduce the risks for other emerging and zoonotic diseases.

Acknowledgements

The authors acknowledge support from the Australian Centre for International Agricultural Research, the Australian Agency for International Development, the Food and Agriculture Organization of the United Nations, the Deutsche Gesellschaft für Technische Zusammenarbeit GmbH, the International Livestock Research Institute, the International Rural Poultry Centre of the Kyeema Foundation, the Universities of Queensland (Australia) and Tufts (USA) and the World Organisation for Animal Health (Office International des Epizooties, OIE). We also extend our gratitude to the veterinarians, extensionists, researchers, traders and livestock producers in many parts of the world who have given freely of their time and expertise over the years.

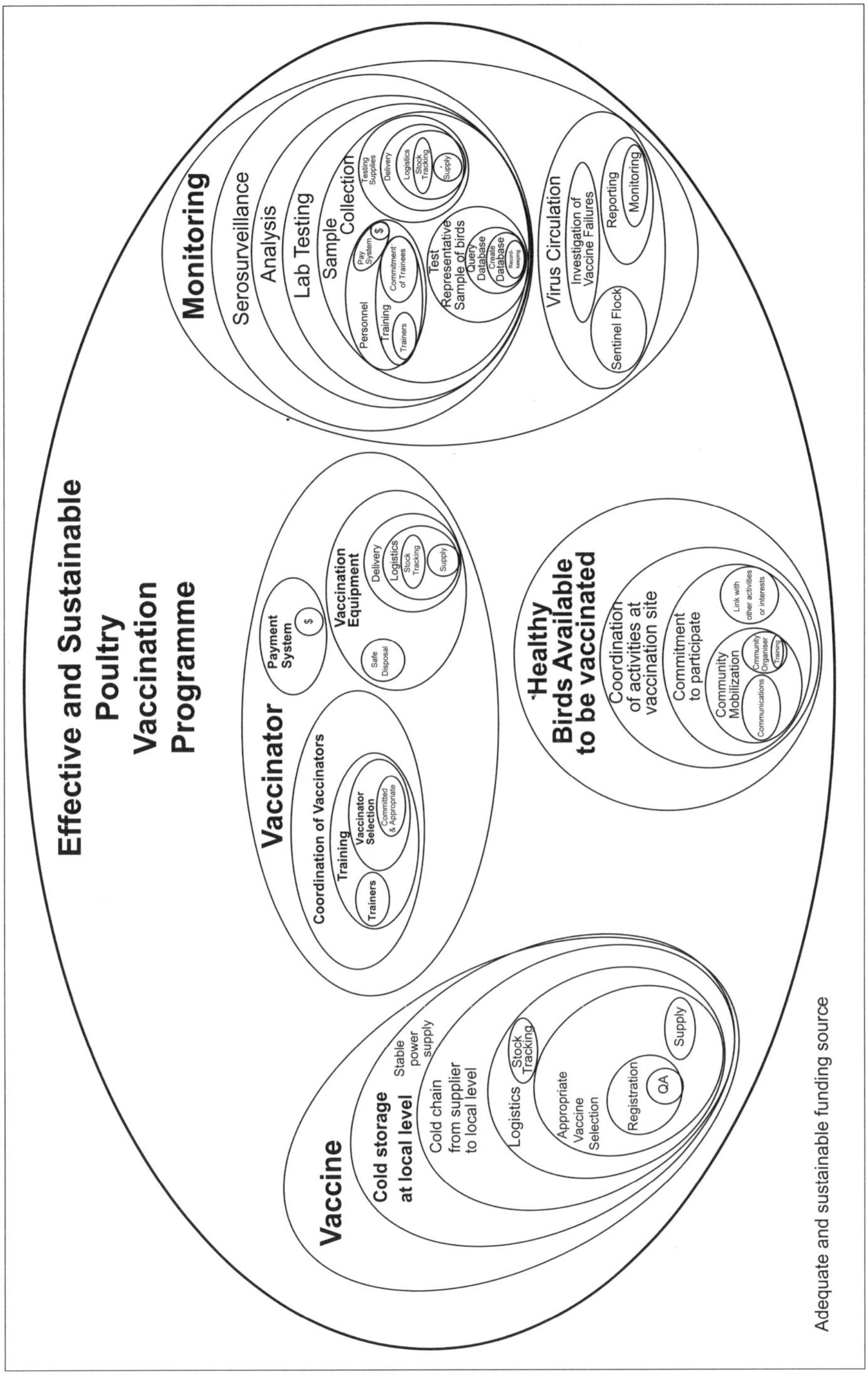

Fig. 1: Components of an effective, sustainable poultry vaccination programme

REFERENCES

1 Zander DV, Bermudez AJ, Mallinson ET: Principles of disease prevention: diagnosis and control. In: Calnek BW, Barnes HJ, Beard CW, McDougald LR, Saif YM, eds, Diseases of Poultry, 10th Ed., London, Mosby-Wolfe, 1997; pp. 3-45.

2 Alexander DJ, Bell JG, Alders RG: Technology review: Newcastle disease with special emphasis on its effect on village chickens (FAO Animal Production and Health Paper No. 161). Rome, Food and Agriculture Organization of the United Nations, 2004.

3 Capua I, Alexander DJ: The challenge of avian influenza to the veterinary community. Avian Pathol 2006, 35:189-205.

4 Alders RG: Sustainable control of Newcastle disease in rural areas. In: Alders RG, Spradbrow PB, eds, SADC Planning Workshop on Newcastle Disease Control in Village Chickens. Proceedings of an International Workshop, Maputo, Mozambique, 6-9 March 2000 (ACIAR Proceedings 103). Canberra, 2001. http://www.aciar.gov.au.

5 Schelling E, Bechir M, Ahmed MA, Wyss, K, Randolph TF, Zinsstag J: Human and animal vaccination delivery to remote nomadic families, Chad. Emerg Infect Dis 2007;13:373-379.

6 Chicamisse M, Harun M, Alders RG, Young MP: Evaluation of the cold chain encountered by 'wet' I-2 Newcastle disease vaccine from the vaccine production department to the village chicken in Mozambique. In: Proceedings of an International Conference, Dar es Salaam, 5-7 October, 2005 (ACIAR Proceedings). Canberra, Australian Centre for International Agricultural Research 2007 (in press).

7 Alders RG, Bagnol B, Young MP: Technically sound and sustainable Newcastle disease control in village chickens: lessons learnt over fifteen years. In: Proceedings of the World's Poultry Science Association Asian Pacific Federation Working Group on Small-scale Family Poultry Farming Symposium, Bangkok, 5-6 March 2007, 2007; pp. 26-33.

8 Anonymous: A joint working paper by participants from Pakistan. In: Asia Productivity Organization Study Meeting on Effective Disease Control and Prevention in the Poultry Sector with Emphasis on Bird Flu, Tehran, 16-21 December 2006.

9 Alders RG, Bagnol B: Effective communication: the key to effective communication: the key to efficient HPAI prevention and control. Worlds Poult Sci J 2007;63:139-147.

10 Viscarra RE, Chipana O, Rushton J: Identifying and meeting the veterinary education needs of poor isolated communities in Bolivia. In: Proceedings of the International Society for Veterinary Epidemiology and Economics, Cairns, 6-11 August 2006. Queensland, Australian College of Veterinary Scientists, Epidemiology Chapter, 2006.

11 McLeod A, Rushton J, Riviere-Cinnamond, A, Brandenburg B, Hinrichs J, Loth L: Economic issues in vaccination against highly pathogenic avian influenza in developing countries. Dev Biol (Basel) 2007;131:63-72

Dr. Robyn Alders, International Rural Poultry Centre, Kyeema Foundation, G.P.O. Box 3023, Brisbane 4001, Australia
E-mail: robyna@kyeemafoundation.org and robyn.alders@gmail.com

Dodet B and the Scientific & Technical Department of the OIE (eds): Vaccination: A Tool for the Control of Avian Influenza. Dev Biol (Basel). Basel, Karger, 2007, vol 130, p 83.

SESSION IV

Application of Vaccination

Chairperson: *G. Brückner,* OIE, France

Dodet B and the Scientific & Technical Department of the OIE (eds): Vaccination: A Tool for the Control of Avian Influenza. Dev Biol (Basel). Basel, Karger, 2007, vol 130, p 85.

Needs Assessment for the Use of Vaccination

M. Weijtens[1], H. Maurice[1], H. Van Langen[1], G. Koch[2]

[1] Ministry of Agriculture, Nature and Food Quality, The Netherlands

[2] Centre for Infectious Disease Control, The Netherlands

Vaccination can be a tool in the prevention, control and eradication of infectious diseases. Emergency vaccination in case of outbreaks of highly pathogenic avian influenza (HPAI) is currently not considered appropriate in the Dutch situation. The Netherlands have however gained experience in preventive vaccination of poultry against Avian Influenza type H5N1. It concerned preventive vaccination of poultry at risk of infection by migrating wild birds: free-range commercial laying hens and so-called hobby poultry. Vaccination was an alternative for compulsory confinement of the poultry.

The Netherlands have applied the following conditions for vaccination:

- the use of an inactivated heterologous vaccine
- identification and registration of all vaccinated poultry
- movement control of vaccinated poultry
- 100% monitoring of the vaccinated flocks for possible introduction of the virus
- monitoring of the efficacy of vaccination (antibody response to vaccination).

Some 8 commercial poultry farmers and 1800 hobby poultry keepers participated in this pilot project. Participation was rather limited due to the fear of problems with the marketing of the eggs (commercial laying hens), and the costs of vaccination and heavy administrative burden (hobby poultry).

No introduction of virus in vaccinated populations was registered, even if the antibody response was not 100% satisfactory.

Dr. Martijn Weijtens, Ministry of Agriculture, Nature and Food Quality, Bezuidenhoutseweg 73 Den Haag, 2500 EK, The Netherlands
E-mail: m.j.b.m.weijtens@minlnv.nl

Dodet B and the Scientific & Technical Department of the OIE (eds): Vaccination: A Tool for the Control of Avian Influenza. Dev Biol (Basel). Basel, Karger, 2007, vol 130, pp 87-97.

Risk Modelling for Vaccination: a Risk Assessment Perspective

M. Wooldridge

Centre for Epidemiology and Risk Analysis, Veterinary Laboratories Agency, New Haw, Addlestone, Surrey, England

Key words: vaccine hazards, vaccine risks, risk assessment, risk modelling

Summary: Any risk assessment involves a number of steps. First, the risk manager, in close liaison with the risk assessor, should identify the question of interest. Then, the hazards associated with each risk question should be identified. Only then can the risks themselves be assessed. Several questions may reasonably be asked about the risk associated with avian influenza vaccines and their use. Some apply to any vaccine, while others are specific to avian influenza. Risks may occur during manufacture and during use. Some concern the vaccines themselves, while others address the effect of failure on disease control. The hazards associated with each risk question are then identified. These may be technical errors in design, development or production, such as contamination or failure to inactivate appropriately. They may relate to the biological properties of the pathogens themselves displayed during manufacture or use, for example, reversion to virulence, shedding or not being the right strain for the subsequent challenge. Following a consideration of risks and hazards, the information needed and an outline of the steps necessary to assess the risk is summarized, for an illustrative risk question using, as an example, the risks associated with the use of vaccines in the field. A brief consideration of the differences between qualitative and quantitative risk assessments is also included, and the potential effects of uncertainty and variability on the results are discussed.

Introduction

Any risk assessment involves a number of steps. First, the risk manager, in close liaison with the risk assessor, should identify the risk questions of interest. Then, the hazards associated with the risk questions should be identified. Only then can the risks themselves be assessed. This process is necessary for any risk assessment, including assessment of risks associated with a vaccine. Below, I briefly describe some key concepts and definitions relevant to risk assessment, and summarize the main hazards and risks in vaccine design and production. The hazards and risks of vaccine use in the field are then described in more detail, and key points are discussed and summarized.

Key Concepts and Definitions

Hazard and risk

Two key concepts in risk assessment are those of 'hazard' and 'risk'. As well as their meanings in everyday usage, there are a variety of specific definitions for each, used within the risk assessment world. In this paper, in the context of vaccination, 'hazard' is defined as a substance or action that may cause harm or an adverse event, and 'risk' is the probability that the hazard will give rise to some harm or adverse event.

Variability and uncertainty

Two other key concepts are variability and uncertainty. In risk assessment, 'variability' is generally taken to mean real life differences, in, for example the weight range of a flock of chickens or differences in the immune response of individual birds. 'Uncertainty' is used to describe situations in which the real value (or range of values, if variability exists) is unknown. In theory, uncertainty can be reduced by further observation and data collection, but this is often not possible in practice or, for rare events, might take many years. Therefore, in many risk assessments, these concepts should be taken into account in estimates and described in the results.

Qualitative and quantitative risk assessments

Risk assessments are often categorized as qualitative or quantitative. A third category is sometimes used, that of semiquantitative risk assessment. Although the terminology and detail may differ, the underlying principles of risk assessment remain the same, whatever codes or guidelines are used. I shall not go into great detail about the methodology of risk assessment or differences between qualitative and quantitative risk assessment, and other texts should be consulted if required. For example, Murray et al. [1], and Wooldridge [2] describe principles and methods for qualitative risk assessments, whereas Murray et al. [3] and Vose [4] address quantitative risk assessments.

The main difference between qualitative and quantitative risk assessment is the form of output or results. In a qualitative risk assessment, the assessment of the risk is presented in text format, as a logical deduction or series of logical deductions based on conclusions from the data collected. The risk is often described as 'high', 'medium', 'low' or 'negligible'. When there is much uncertainty or variability, however, even this level of conclusion may not be possible. In these cases, a logical description of the major conclusions is given, including a description of the degree of uncertainty or variability [2]. Quantitative risk assessments are those in which the final risk estimate is numerical, given either as a single point value or as a distribution, depending on the method used. Deterministic models give point values, whereas stochastic models are often used in the presence of uncertainty, to allow for a risk estimate that takes this into account mathematically. Semi-quantitative risk assessments generally use categories to describe the risk estimate results. For a number of methodological reasons, such estimates should be used and interpreted with care, and, for that reason, their use can be controversial. Nevertheless, they are often used to rank or set priorities on risks, and may be useful for that purpose.

The risk question

The risk question is the specific question that is used as the basis of a risk assessment. It should be agreed between the risk manager and the risk assessor before the risk assessment is begun in order that the risk assessor knows precisely which risks are of interest to the risk manager, and the risk manager knows precisely which risk estimates he or she will eventually receive. In practice, it might be necessary to revisit and rephrase the risk question during the work, again with discussion and agreement between the assessor and the manager. In any risk assessment, the final risk question must be specific, but this is especially crucial for a quantitative risk assessment, in which, for example, a time frame or an equivalent (e.g. risk per year or risk per individual animal) should be specified. For any issue, including vaccines, many potential risk questions can be asked, and a number of risk assessments might have to be undertaken on different aspects, with different risk questions. Examples are considered below.

Hazards and Risks Associated with Vaccine Design and Production

Hazards in design and production

A number of aims and requirements must be taken into account in designing a vaccine. For example, the way in which a given vaccine is intended to act can vary: it might be intended primarily to prevent infection of the vaccinated animal, or it might be intended primarily to prevent clinical signs, i.e. disease. For either intention, a level of efficacy must be reached in the final design that makes its production and use worthwhile, although efficacy is highly unlikely ever to reach 100% on an individual animal basis. Vaccines can be produced from live attenuated or inactivated virus; to achieve acceptable levels of efficacy, various adjuvants may be included. An additional aim might be to ensure that vaccinated animals can be differentiated from infected animals. Vaccines made from an antigen that is only a small part of the virus can help to achieve this aim. There are thus a variety of general hazards connected with these features which may affect the efficacy of the vaccine - and therefore also the risk (or probability) of failure to be effective, and also the probability to cause harm. With a virus group that includes many strains or which mutates rapidly, such as avian influenza virus, there are additional problems in design. The design stage must include a decision on which strain or strains should be used to give the most appropriate protection in the defined population of interest. Design of the commercial production process is also a part of vaccine design.

When designing and producing a vaccine and assessing the risks in the design and production process, a complete list must be drawn up of the potential hazards that might cause the vaccine to fail to act in the way intended. At the design stage, these hazards can be categorized into those associated with inappropriate design of the vaccine itself and those associated with inappropriate design of the production process when scaling-up for commercial manufacture. There are also hazards associated with the production process, such as those that will prevent the vaccine from meeting production and quality standards and requirements. Identification of the full range of hazards associated with vaccine design and production and their potential effects requires close liaison between the risk assessor and those responsible for vaccine design and production. Examples of potential hazards in vaccine design and production are given in Table 1.

Table 1: Examples of potential hazards in vaccine design and production

Hazards in design	**Hazards in production**
Main aim(s) of vaccine not considered	Contamination of vaccine with other biological agents
Selection of poorly antigenic virus or strain	Presence of other (non-infectious) contaminants in the vaccine
Selection of wrong virus strain for prevalent field infections	Low titre or antigen content
Poor choice of antigen type, e.g. inactivated, live attenuated, subunit, recombinant	Overpotent (titre of live agent too high)
Failure to allow differentiation of vaccinated animals from infected animals (DIVA)	Incomplete inactivation or attenuation (as appropriate)
Ineffective adjuvant	Incorrect or missing (multivalent vaccines) vaccine strain
Instability of product, leading to e.g. reduced efficacy, mutation of virus in use, vaccine spread to non-target species	Test results (e.g. pH) different from specification
	Failure of quality control system
	Contamination of production workers with virulent pathogen
	Escape of virulent pathogen from production plant

Risk assessment in vaccine design and production

The key risk question in vaccine design and production is likely to be: "What is the probability that this vaccine, at the point of dispatch from the manufacturer, will not be, or will not function, as intended?" This risk question covers such issues as efficacy, stability, physical properties, contamination and any other intended properties. In order to attempt to ensure that the vaccine is, and functions as, intended certain risk reduction measures (safeguards) are used, including testing of the vaccine in clinical trials to assess safety and efficacy, quality control and specification testing (integral to good manufacturing practice (GMP)), plant biosecurity and post-release pharmacovigilance. Most of these activities are also integral to authorization or licensing.

In clinical trials conducted as part of the design and production process, vaccinated animals will undergo challenge in controlled conditions, both experimental and 'field', to assess the risk that it will not behave in use as it was intended to do by design. The information produced will be quantitative data giving a comparison of the intended with the actual behaviour of the vaccine in these tests. Ideally, the testing regime is planned such that quantitative estimates of comparison can be obtained for any aspect of intended behaviour, and in particular for efficacy in preventing infection or preventing or reducing clinical signs, as appropriate.

Once suitable test data have been obtained, the risk assessor can assess the probability that the vaccine conforms to specified standards and the probability that it will fail to behave as intended. Only a limited number of scenarios can be tested before a vaccine is released onto the market, however, whereas an infinite number of scenarios can occur in conditions of actual use.

Thus, vaccines released for use would usually be:

- authorized for production and use, with demonstrated efficacy and safety if used as directed;
- quality controlled in production, with a known failure rate, and failed batches held back;
- and have data available allowing an assessment, potentially quantitative, of risks if used as directed and under the specified conditions.

Hazards and Risks Associated with Vaccine Use under Field Conditions

Hazards in field use

Risk assessment becomes more difficult in the field. Some key issues for use of avian influenza vaccine in the field include the risks that the vaccine will not act as intended in preventing infection and disease in vaccinated birds, in preventing further spread of virus to which the vaccinated flock is exposed, and in its safety to target and non-target species. These risks are the result of hazards in the field which lead to use of the vaccine in ways not specified in the licensing process. Some examples of potential hazards are given in Table 2.

Table 2: Examples of potential hazards in field use of vaccines

Vaccine not properly maintained before use e.g. no cold chain (if required), out of date
Vaccine delivery poorly executed e.g. wrong site or tissue, failure to inject, contaminated needle
Wrong type of vaccine selected or accidentally given
Vaccine and field virus strains different
Vaccine given after infection
Variability of immune system in vaccinated population leading to poor response
Vaccine contaminated in use
Species vaccinated not that for which vaccine was designed or licensed, leading to poor response

Risk assessment in field use of vaccines

The major risk reduction measures (safeguards) in the field are knowledge and understanding of those handling and using the vaccines and, on the basis of that knowledge, the care they take in handling and use, plus the level of facilities and resources available in the field. These safeguards are 'soft' and much more variable than those in the design and production stages, and there are unlikely to be hard data on many of them to allow a quantitative assessment of risks associated with field use. A risk assessment is still useful, however, for identifying risk pathways, which are useful in themselves, and identifying also the specific data needed for further assessment.

The best way to illustrate a practical approach to undertaking such a risk assessment is to use a specific example. For this illustration, it is assumed that the risk question agreed with the risk manager is: "What is the probable efficacy of vaccine V in preventing infection in flock F under conditions of field use?" For this vaccine, the efficacy indicated by the authorization is defined as EA, and the risk question makes the implicit assumption that the conditions in field use might not be ideal. As in any risk assessment, the initial step is to identify the steps in the risk pathway, or model 'backbone'. This is frequently an iterative process and the usual practice of the risk assessor cross-checking this pathway with appropriate experts should be undertaken (here for example avian influenza vaccine experts).

Taking the example risk question above, in order that the efficacy is not reduced from that in the authorisation process (EA), the conditions which must be met (steps, S) and which comprise the risk pathway are given in Table 3. If, at any step, these conditions are not met, a change of efficacy (usually a reduction) is likely, and any reduction is an unwanted outcome, the risk of which is being assessed. For each of the steps shown in Table 3, there is a probability of the specified conditions not being met, which will result, as indicated previously, in a change (probably a reduction) in efficacy at each step, giving a final efficacy for vaccine V in field use (E_{use}).

Table 3: Steps in the risk pathway for the risk question: "What is the probable efficacy of vaccine V in preventing infection in flock F under field use conditions?"

Step in risk pathway	Description of step
S1	Assume that the design efficiency, EA, of vaccine V, at the point of production, is as assessed at authorization.
S2	Vaccine V is kept under conditions as directed until use.
S3	Vaccine V is administered as directed.
S4	Flock F has the same overall immune response as the flocks used in authorization testing.
S5	Flock F is exposed to the strain of virus that vaccine V is intended for use against.

Table 4 summarizes the effect of the probability P that the required conditions are not met at any stage (defined here as PS2, PS3, PS4, and PS5). Therefore, in order to assess fully the effect of failure to meet the required conditions at each step, one must be able to estimate the probability that the required conditions for that step will not be met and the probable effect on efficacy. Figure 1 shows, diagrammatically, the effects of the probabilities listed in Table 4.

Table 4: Summary of the effect on efficacy of vaccine V by failure to meet required conditions at each stage of risk pathway for field use

Step in risk pathway	Probability that required conditions are not met at each stage	Probable effect on efficacy
S1	Assumption: Vaccine V is at point of retail, therefore it has assessed (design) efficacy **EA** as per authorisation process	Assumed to be **EA** (i.e. it is assumed vaccine complies with authorisation standards)
S2	Probability that vaccine V is not kept as directed until use: **PS2**	EA is reduced to **E2** by poor storage conditions
S3	Probability that vaccine V is not administered as directed: **PS3**	E2 is reduced to **E3** by incorrect administration
S4	Probability that flock F has a different (maybe better or worse) overall immune response than the flocks used in authorisation testing: **PS4**	Where flock F has, overall, an immune response which is less good than flocks used in testing, E3 is reduced to **E4** (and vice versa)
S5	Probability that flock F is exposed to a different strain of virus to that which vaccine V is intended for use against: **PS5**	E4 is reduced to $\mathbf{E_{use}}$ as challenged with different strain

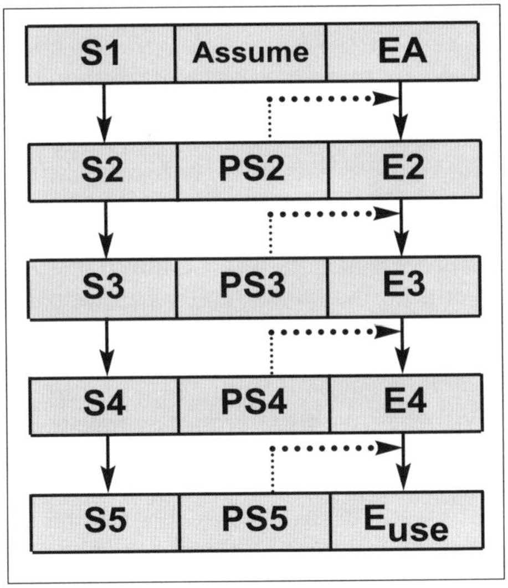

Fig. 1: Steps in the risk pathway (S1–S5), the probability that the required conditions at each step will not be met (PS2–PS5) and their cumulative effect on the probable efficacy of vaccine V in field use (E_{use}) for the risk question defined in the text

The next step in undertaking this risk assessment is to collect data on the probable effect if the required ('ideal') conditions are not met at each step, and data to assess the probable effect on efficacy of each change from ideal conditions. Table 5 summarizes the 'ideal' data needed for this assessment, assuming that the value of EA is known from data obtained during authorization and licensing. The usual place to start finding data is the published literature; however, for risk assessments, raw data are generally best, so it may often be necessary to try and go back to the authors of published results for this. Unpublished data from those working in the field are another potential source of data. However, there are many potential problems in collecting data for such risk assessments.

Table 5: Summary of the data needs for each step in the risk pathway (given that data for step 1, the value of EA, is known)

Step	Data on probability of	Data on the effect on efficacy of
S2	Vaccines not being kept as directed until use (PS2)	Failure to keep vaccine V as directed
S3	Vaccines not administered as directed (PS3)	Incorrect administration of vaccine V
S4	Overall immune response of field flocks being different from that of trial flocks (and range of responses) (PS4)	The range of overall immune responses across flocks
S5	Flock F being exposed to a different strain of virus to that which Vaccine V is intended for use against (PS5)	Vaccine V being used against other strains of virus than those intended in authorization process

To obtain the value for EA, the manufacturer and licensing authorities would be the places to start. However, is the initial assumption that the vaccine has the quoted efficacy EA, at the point of supply from the manufacturer, likely to be correct? This may depend upon where the vaccine was manufactured, and under what practical conditions and legal controls. For vaccines manufactured in response to an emergency situation, in less than ideal practical conditions in remote regions, it may not always be the case. It is also very likely that data will be lacking on actual conditions of vaccine storage under field conditions, on the skill and care of administration in the field and on the immunity status (on average and by range) of the flocks targeted for vaccination. While there may be some data on probable challenge strains obtained from surveillance activities, they cannot be predicted with certainty until a challenge occurs. Thus there is likely to be much uncertainty present in any data available and, even when 'good' data are available, there will be variability. The data on the effect of actual conditions on efficacy are likely to be restricted to a limited number of scenarios used during testing and clinical trials. Thus, there are likely to be many data gaps for this risk assessment. Table 6 indicates some of the ways in which the necessary data might be obtained.

An alternative source of information routinely used for risk assessments is expert opinion. This involves the selection of appropriate experts and elicitation of estimates of the missing information, including, for quantitative risk assessments, the model parameters. There are many issues in the use of experts, including their selection, the methods used to obtain their opinions (for example, questionnaires and workshops, often based on the Delphi method), minimizing bias and conversion to numerical values. When hard data are scarce, however, and pragmatic assessment results are required by the risk manager, expert opinion is often the only alternative (for an example, see [5]) and may be necessary until better data become available. When data are scarce, uncertain or variable, which is likely to be the case in risk assessments of field use of vaccine, it is essential to ensure that the variability and uncertainty is reflected in the resultant risk estimates. The method depends on whether the risk assessment is qualitative or quantitative. Once the risk question has been agreed, the risk pathway described and the data collected, the risk of interest (here, the probable reduction in efficacy of the vaccine in field use) is assessed. As indicated earlier, appropriate texts should be consulted for methodological details of the conduct of risk assessments, both qualitative and quantitative. In brief, for qualitative risk assessments, all the data used are documented in a logical order corresponding to the steps in the risk pathway, and logical deductions are made about the risk at each step and, if possible, about the overall risk. In the risk question considered here, the assessed likely outcome might be, for example, 'a negligible reduction in efficacy' or 'a very great reduction in efficacy' or another appropriate conclusion, depending on the data. As also noted earlier, the text must also describe the uncertainty and variability within the data and their effect on the final risk estimate. For quantitative risk assessments, all data, including expert opinion, are converted into model parameters, and a mathematical model based on the risk pathway is used with the appropriate mathematical methods to calculate a numerical description of the reduction in efficacy. In this case, uncertainty and variability are also described mathematically, with distributions used as inputs to the model and to describe the final risk estimate.

Table 6: Potential ways of obtaining the necessary data for vaccine field use risk assessments

Data required to estimate	**Potential methods of data collection**
Probability of conditions of storage and use	Observational field studies
Probability of flock differences (in terms of e.g. breed, age structure, disease status) and their effect on overall flock immune status and response	Knowledge of (and data on) the poultry industry in the region of interest to determine probable flock characteristicsExperimental work to determine effect of flock characteristics on overall immune status and response
Probability that challenge strain is different from that for which the vaccine was designed	Local, regional and worldwide surveillance of viral spread by strain
Probable effect of any of the above factors on efficacy of vaccine in field use	Results of experimental challenge Results of outbreak field studies

Key Points in Modelling the Risks of Vaccination

Assessments of the risks in the design and production of vaccine are routinely undertaken for authorization and licensing requirements. These result in directions for use on the basis of data obtained in tests and clinical trials. Experimental and trial work on the full range of potential field conditions would, however, be impractical and probably impossible. In field use, resources and practical conditions often mean that directions are not, or cannot be, followed and this failure is likely to affect the efficacy of the vaccine. Risk assessments for field use of a vaccine might therefore be required, as illustrated above. Field use risk assessments are difficult to undertake, however, as shown in Table 7.

Table 7: Comparison of the key differences likely to be found in risk assessments for the design and production stages of vaccine manufacture compared with those undertaken for field use.

Risk assessments for design and production of vaccines	Risk assessments for field use of vaccines
Data rich: from experimental work, physical tests, clinical trials	Data poor: many gaps (uncertainty), real life variability, expert opinion used
Good safeguards: controlled process, good manufacturing practice (GMP), quality control, licensing	Poor safeguards: reliance on knowledge, care and local resources
Risk assessments relatively easy	Risk assessments complex and difficult

Given the lack of data and the complexity and difficulty of undertaking risk assessments for vaccine use in the field, one might ask whether results obtained with so much uncertainty and variability are meaningful - particularly since decisions on their use are frequently based on other factors. However, frequently the main reason for undertaking risk assessments it to give insights into the processes occurring which affect the outcome, for example an elucidation of the precise chain of events necessary for particular outcomes (the risk pathways) and/or the identification of crucial data deficiencies. This allows for targeted data collection, from experimental or observational field studies, as appropriate, which will improve the data available and thus the overall risk estimate. Explicit identification of the full range of risk pathways also allows for the incorporation of risk reduction measures ('safeguards') into those risk pathways, even before more data become available thus avoiding redundant controls which will not affect the risk at all. Although further data collection will not reduce variability, the identification and source of the variability is useful for risk management. Finally, even though the use of vaccines is often based on other factors (including 'political' and trade considerations), improving risk assessments and predictions of effects in field use are likely, in turn, to eventually have an influence on those other factors.

References

1 Murray N, MacDiarmid S, Wooldridge M, Gummow B, Morley R, Weber S, Giovannini A, Wilson D: Handbook on Import Risk Analysis for Animals and their Products. Volume 1. Introduction and Qualitative Risk Analysis. Paris, World Organisation for Animal Health, 2004.

2 Wooldridge M: Qualitative risk assessment. In: Schaffner D, ed. Microbial Risk Analysis in Foods. Washington DC, American Society for Microbiology, 2007/pp.1-29.

3 Murray N, MacDiarmid S, Wooldridge M, Gummow B, Morley R, Weber S, Giovannini A, Wilson D: Handbook on Import Risk Analysis for Animals and their Products. Volume 2. Quantitative Risk Analysis. Paris, World Organisation for Animal Health, 2004.

4 Vose D: Risk Analysis: A Quantitative Guide. Chichester, John Wiley & Sons, 2000.

5 Gallagher E, Ryan J, Kelly L, Leforban Y, Wooldridge M: Estimating the risk of importation of foot-and-mouth disease into Europe. Vet Rec 2002;150:769-772.

Prof. Marion Wooldridge, Centre for Epidemiology and Risk Analysis, Veterinary Laboratories Agency, New Haw, Addlestone, KT15 3NB
E-mail: m.wooldridge@vla.defra.gsi.gov.uk

Dodet B and the Scientific & Technical Department of the OIE (eds): Vaccination: A Tool for the Control of Avian Influenza. Dev Biol (Basel). Basel, Karger, 2007, vol 130, pp 99-108.

Planning and Executing a Vaccination Campaign against Avian Influenza

S. Marangon, A. Cristalli, L. Busani

Istituto Zooprofilattico delle Venezie, Legnaro (Padova), Italy

Keywords: avian influenza, HPAI, LPAI, vaccination campaign

Summary: Vaccination against avian influenza infection caused by H5 or H7 virus subtypes has been used on several occasions in recent years to control and in some cases eradicate the disease. In order to contain avian influenza infection effectively, immunization should be combined with a coordinated set of control and monitoring measures. The outcome of an immunization campaign depends on the territorial strategy; whereas the capacity of the veterinary services in developed countries permits enforcement of strategies aimed at eradicating avian influenza, many countries currently affected by highly pathogenic avian influenza (HPAI) H5N1 viruses have a limited veterinary infrastructure and a limited capacity to respond to such epidemics. In these countries, resources are still insufficient to conduct adequate surveillance for identification and reaction to avian influenza outbreaks when they occur. When properly applied in this scenario, immunization can reduce mortality and production losses. In the long term, immunization might also decrease the prevalence of infection to levels at which stamping-out and surveillance can be applied. Countries should adapt their immunization programmes to local conditions in order to guarantee their efficacy and sustainability. In the initial emergency phase, human resources can be mobilized, with reliance on personal responsibility and motivation, thus compensating for potential shortcomings in organization. A more appropriate allocation of resources must be pursued in the long term, remembering that biosecurity is the main component of an exit strategy and must always be improved.

INTRODUCTION

Control of avian influenza has become more complex than in the past. The unprecedented worldwide spread of these infections and the related serious animal and human health implications have made it necessary to develop control strategies that are alternatives or complementary to the stamping-out policy that has usually been used to control and eradicate this disease. In view of the high risk for major epidemics of avian influenza once the viruses have been introduced into domestic poultry populations, alternatives are needed to stamping-out in the case of outbreaks of H5 and H7 of low-pathogenicity (LPAI) or highly pathogenic avian influenza (HPAI). Control can be achieved by a combination of biosecurity, stamping-out, restriction and immunization. While the capacity of the veterinary services in developed countries permits enforcement of a strategy aimed at eradicating avian influenza, many of the countries currently affected by H5N1 HPAI viruses have inadequate veterinary infrastructures and resources to conduct adequate surveillance for diagnosis and response. If properly applied in this scenario, immunization can reduce poultry mortality and production losses and safeguard food supplies and livelihoods. In developing countries, the aim of vaccination is to control an epidemic in the short term, at the same time decreasing the prevalence of infection to a level at which an eradication strategy could be implemented in the long term. Adaptation of avian influenza vaccination programmes to local situations is a prerequisite for their efficacy and sustainability.

We describe the planning of an avian influenza vaccination campaign and discuss its organization and execution, while at the same time considering the major limitations and drawbacks of this disease control policy.

Vaccination for the Control of Avian Influenza

Experimental and field data have shown that vaccination can be a valuable option for avian influenza control [1]. Vaccination against avian influenza viruses, including H5N1 HPAI, has been proven to be effective in chickens, geese and ducks under both experimental conditions and in the field [2,3]. In turkeys challenged with various low-pathogenicity virus subtypes, the infectious dose needed to infect vaccinated birds was significantly higher than that for sham controls, and a significant reduction in virus shedding was observed [4]. The results of challenge and transmission experiments indicate that, although vaccination cannot always avoid infection, it provides protection against disease signs and death. The increase in infectious dose needed to infect vaccinated birds and the decrease in the amount and duration of virus shedding reduce the transmission level to that at which a major outbreak can be prevented [5,6].

Vaccines have been used to control epidemics of avian influenza due to both low and highly pathogenic forms in several countries (Table 1), showing that the disease can be controlled and eradicated [7]. This experience indicates that immunization combined with a territorial control strategy is effective for the management and control of avian influenza infections.

Vaccination Programmes in Various Scenarios

Before an avian influenza immunization campaign is initiated, a well-defined plan of the main activities and the vaccination programme suited to local production systems must be prepared, with particular attention to critical aspects that might affect the outcome. Generally, an emergency vaccination programme should include decision-making patterns for various conditions, and it should be defined in the framework of the national avian influenza contingency plan. In particular, a vaccination strategy must be defined and a decision taken about whether to target only certain categories of poultry or all susceptible birds. All activities related to the campaign must be defined, organized and applied in relation to the particular situations of different regions, areas or compartments. As avian influenza has occurred in several areas of the world, more than one vaccination scenario should be considered. Application of different vaccination options should also take into account the virus strain involved, the eco-epidemiological situation, the characteristics of the poultry-producing sector, the capacity of the veterinary infrastructure and the availability of adequate resources.

Table 1: Use of immunization to control avian influenza outbreaks due to H5 and H7 subtype viruses

Avian influenza virus	**Country**	**Period**	**Type of vaccine**	**No. of doses (million)**	**Bird species**
HPAI H5N2	Mexico	1995-2001	Inactivated oil emulsion H5N2	1423.1	Broilers, breeders, layers, grandparents
HPAI H5N2	Mexico	1998-2001	Recombinant fowlpox H5	459	Broilers, breeders
LPAI H7N3	Utah (USA)	1995	Inactivated-oil emulsion H7N3	2.0	Turkeys
LPAI H7N2	Connecticut (USA)	2003	Inactivated-oil emulsion H7N3 Inactivated-oil emulsion H7N2	3.2 Not available	Layers
HPAI H5N1	Egypt	2006	Inactivated-oil emulsion H5N2 and H5N1	5.4	Poultry (including backyard)
LPAI H7N3 and LPAI H5N2	Italy	2003-2005	Inactivated-oil emulsion H7N1 Inactivated-oil emulsion H5/H7	75.6 87.2	Turkeys, layers, cockerels, capons
HPAI H7N3	Pakistan	1995-2003	Inactivated-oil emulsion H7N3	Not available	Breeders, grandparents
HPAI H5N1	Pakistan	2006-2007	Inactivated H5N2	Not available	Breeders, poultry (ring vaccination)
HPAI H5N1	Hong Kong	2002-2003	Inactivated-oil emulsion H5N2	0.29	Chicken broilers
HPAI H5N1	Indonesia	2004-2006	H5N1	86	Chickens, ducks
HPAI H5N1	China	2003-2006	Inactivated-oil emulsion H5N2	4880	Ducks, geese, chickens
HPAI H5N1	Viet Nam	2005-2006	Inactivated-oil emulsion H5N2 and H5N1; Live fowl-pox recombinant vaccine	246	Ducks, geese, chickens
HPAI H5N1	Afghanistan	2007	Not available	Not available	Poultry
HPAI H5N1	Russian Federation	2006-2007	Not available	≥ 1	Backyard poultry, small farms
HPAI H5N1	Russian Federation (Siberia)	2006	Not available	10	Poultry
HPAI H5N1	Côte d'Ivoire	2006-2007	Inactivated-oil emulsion H5N9	> 0.2	Backyard and large poultry enterprises

Eco-epidemiological situation

Until 1998, avian influenza was a disease of minor importance, but since 1999 infections have no longer been considered sporadic. If estimates of the ongoing H5N1 HPAI epidemic are included, several hundred million birds have been affected by this disease in the past 8 years. The epidemics in Italy in 1999–2000, The Netherlands in 2003 and Canada in 2004 and the ongoing epidemic of H5N1 HPAI (2003–2007) have had a devastating effect on the poultry production sector and on society as a whole. In some cases, significant human health issues have been created, including the risk for a new pandemic virus for humans through the avian–human link.

In the ecology of avian influenza viruses, HPAI viruses originated from low-pathogenicity viruses of the H5 and H7 subtypes introduced into domestic terrestrial poultry from the wild-bird reservoir. Before the advent of H5N1, none of the HPAI viruses persisted in an endemic fashion in domestic or wild-bird populations. H5N1 HPAI was isolated from herons, egrets, and peregrine falcons in Hong Kong in 2002–2003, indicating that wild birds can be infected and can spread the virus to terrestrial poultry [8]. H5N1 HPAI has been endemic in aquatic poultry populations in southeast China since 1997, and its recent isolation from apparently healthy migratory birds in southern China suggests that they might be responsible for long-distance transmission during migration [9]. If the H5N1 virus behaves like a low-pathogenicity type in wild aquatic birds and becomes endemic in at least some wild migratory species, it could represent a permanent threat to domestic bird populations worldwide.

Poultry sector

The characteristics of poultry production systems are one of the most important variables to be considered, including the size of the population in the affected region, area or compartment, the poultry species and types of production involved, their geographical distribution and the worldwide movement of live birds and poultry products.

The FAO position paper [10] on avian influenza control classifies poultry production in Asia into four sectors on the basis of the level of biosecurity applied, from sector 1 for integrated industrial systems with high biosecurity to sector 4 for village or backyard production with minimal biosecurity. Use of immunization against avian influenza should be evaluated on the basis of the levels of biosecurity in the four sectors and the estimated levels of challenge in each production sector, in order to facilitate decision-making.

Veterinary infrastructure and resource availability

Key points in the use of vaccination for avian influenza control are the level of organization of veterinary services and the availability of adequate laboratory capacity. For several reasons, many developing countries, countries with economies in transition and even some industrialized countries do not have an efficient veterinary infrastructure. Shortages of materials, equipment and financial resources also limit the ability to implement a vaccination programme promptly and to put in place sustainable, long-term control measures, such as vaccination, surveillance, early detection of disease and restrictions. The availability of resources for a vaccination campaign is critical, as dedicated economic support, operational research techniques and appropriate facilities for management and communication are essential. Several initiatives are under way to put avian influenza on the development agenda of the most affected regions by raising awareness, mobilizing finances, building capacity and sharing knowledge. National borders cannot stop avian influenza from spreading; only regional cooperation is likely to achieve success in controlling the disease.

Vaccination Strategies for Controlling Avian Influenza

Depending on the eco-epidemiological situation in the affected region, area or compartment and the risk for introduction, a number of vaccination strategies could be used to control avian influenza: preventive (i.e. prophylactic) vaccination when there is a high risk for virus incursion, emergency vaccination in the face of an epidemic and routine vaccination in endemic areas [7].

Preventive (prophylactic) vaccination

Preventive vaccination against the H5 and H7 subtypes of avian influenza virus can be considered a temporary measure; it is usually maintained as long as there is a risk for introduction of avian influenza. It can be used in countries with adequate veterinary infrastructures and sufficient resources and should be based on a risk assessment showing a high risk for the introduction and spread of the virus in domestic poultry. The scientific basis for the use of this strategy is to generate protective immunity in the target population, which can be boosted by additional vaccination in the face of an immediate risk or evidence of the introduction of a field virus. With effective biosecurity, preventive vaccination can maximize protection of poultry at high risk for exposure. Use of this strategy should prevent introduction of avian influenza viruses or reduce their spread, minimizing the effects on poultry production and economic losses. In accordance with the epidemiological situation and on the basis of the risk assessment, a bivalent (H5 and H7) or a monovalent (either H5 or H7) vaccine should be used.

Emergency vaccination

Emergency vaccination is an option when there is evidence of the introduction of avian influenza into a region, area or compartment and where massive, rapid spread of infection might occur, for instance:

- in densely populated poultry areas or areas where agricultural conditions, poultry farming practices and environmental factors could favour establishment of endemic status;
- in the face of difficulty in using massive stamping-out measures because of the importance of poultry as a source of income; and
- in other situations, such as when protected birds, zoo birds and rare breed collections or birds kept in protected areas (as pets or in sanctuaries) are threatened.

The efficacy of an emergency vaccination programme depends on the capacity to limit initial spread of the infection during the high-risk period and on rapid implementation of effective field operations, generally related to:

- correct identification of the compartment and the poultry species to be targeted;
- prompt deployment of adequate vaccines; and
- rapid enforcement of appropriate complementary monitoring and control measures.

A specific type of emergency vaccination is 'ring vaccination' in a defined area around an outbreak in order to bring the outbreak under control as quickly as possible. If promptly implemented, this strategy can help contain the spread of infection.

Routine vaccination

Routine vaccination is the last resort when avian influenza is endemic and adequate measures to contain and eradicate it cannot be enforced due to local conditions. This strategy is probably unsustainable in the long term and in large areas, and, without any additional intervention, will not lead to the eradication of infection because of the difficulty of inducing and maintaining a high level of immune protection in a large poultry population for an extended time. Nevertheless, when used properly, it can reduce mortality and production losses. In the long term, it can also decrease susceptible poultry populations and the prevalence of infection, with possible extension of disease-free compartments and areas. Eventually, long-term vaccination programmes should either be adapted and more closely targeted for greater sustainability or interrupted, provided that contingency plans can be applied to deal with possible re-emergence of the disease.

Mass or targeted vaccination

Immunization can be applied to all susceptible birds in the area (mass vaccination) or to defined species and categories of poultry (targeted vaccination). The choice should be based on a risk analysis that includes an assessment of the susceptibility of the different poultry species, the biosecurity levels of the holdings, the value of the flocks and the risk for disease introduction [11]. Domestic poultry, such as turkeys, are susceptible to both the low- and high-pathogenicity forms of avian influenza. Wild waterfowl, which are the natural reservoir of the viruses, carry and transmit the infection to domestic birds. Domestic waterfowl show relative resistance to the clinical disease caused by H5N1 HPAI, and they could act as carriers of the HPAI virus, thus allowing the infection to persist and spread. Rural duck flocks have been shown to play a role in keeping H5N1 HPAI in circulation in South-East Asia, and specific measures, including vaccination, are being used in this compartment [12].

Factors to be Considered in Planning and Executing a Vaccination Campaign Against Avian Influenza

Certain logistical factors and constraints can significantly influence the outcome of a vaccination campaign and should be taken into account for adequate planning and execution of a field intervention. At the beginning of a vaccination campaign, an overall cost-benefit analysis should be performed, taking into account the economic impact of restriction and biosecurity measures and the implications for trade. The costs of vaccines, vaccine delivery, surveillance, laboratory testing and all other aspects of vaccination must also be considered. A decision to use vaccination to combat avian influenza should be taken promptly after the risk assessment, while also considering the potential implications for human health. Risk assessment also allows correct identification of the region, area or compartment in which vaccination should be applied. The duration of the programme should be defined in advance, bearing in mind its sustainability.

Characteristics, composition and availability of vaccines

Many vaccines against avian influenza have been developed and tested under experimental conditions, but only inactivated whole avian influenza virus vaccines and an H5–avian influenza–recombinant virus-vectored fowlpox vaccine have been licensed and used in the field. Use of these vaccines in a vaccination programme is, however, labour-intensive as both require administration to individual birds. The inactivated vaccine can induce protection in several species of bird, but in order to ensure high levels of immune protection in poultry with long production cycles (e.g. layers, breeders and turkeys), more than one administration is needed. The recombinant virus-vectored fowlpox vaccine can be used only in chickens [13]. New vaccines are being evaluated, and reverse genetics-derived H5-inactivated vaccines have shown promising results in protecting chickens, ducks and geese against H5N1 challenge [2,14]. Vaccine quality should be guaranteed: manufacturers must respect quality standards issued by international bodies in order to ensure high-quality products, and quality certification from regulatory and independent institutions should be obtained before widespread field use.

Vaccine availability is one of the most important variables in prompt application of vaccination against avian influenza. When a new vaccine has to be produced (e.g. introduction/circulation of a new virus strain in domestic poultry), the time required for production can take 4–8 months. Therefore, the number of doses needed to implement and sustain vaccination should be evaluated carefully. Vaccine banks for emergency vaccination should be set up and maintained and based on continuous surveillance of the antigenic characteristics of the viruses in circulation.

Vaccine delivery

Due consideration must be given to the logistics of vaccine delivery in different scenarios. The most suitable vaccine delivery system must be identified and organized, taking into account the problems involved in vaccinating large numbers of birds one by one. Vaccination crews are generally used, with appropriate biosecurity and hygienic measures to reduce the risk for further spread of infection from uncontrolled movements of people. Vaccines should be administered by trained personnel following the recommended protocols. The level of cooperation of poultry producers and vaccine field staff can be increased by raising awareness of the importance of the disease and the losses it can engender. Particularly in the case of a mass vaccination campaign involving all poultry-producing sectors, every resource should be mobilized to promote greater awareness and participation of the community as a whole.

The vaccine delivery system significantly affects the outcome of immunization. Storage and transport are critical factors in vaccine efficacy and should meet the manufacturers' recommendations scrupulously.

Once the type of vaccine to be used has been decided, the vaccination schedules for different bird species and production types (route of administration, number and timing of vaccinations) should be defined to ensure use of the most efficient protocols to obtain the best results in the field, such as blocking virus transmission. If the vaccine schedule is modified with respect to established practice or the manufacturers' instructions (e.g. bird species different from those listed on the fact sheet, different administration schemes), the efficacy of the vaccination scheme should be tested in advance under field conditions before wider application.

Territorial strategy

Experience in the use of vaccines against H5 and H7 indicates that vaccination must be part of a wider territorial strategy to control infection. Essentially, a territorial strategy aims to:

- ensure adequate implementation of the vaccination campaign;
- monitor evolution of the infection and vaccine efficacy;
- detect and adequately manage avian influenza outbreaks; and
- enforce appropriate biosecurity, restriction and control measures.

To improve the efficacy of a vaccination campaign, additional monitoring and control measures should be undertaken and adapted to the capacity of the veterinary infrastructure and the characteristics of the poultry-producing sector in the countries affected. Post-vaccination monitoring and surveillance are essential. Countries with strong veterinary services should monitor the level of immune protection and possible evolution of the infection in the vaccinated population. These activities could be based on use of a suitable discriminatory test or on inspection and testing of unvaccinated sentinel birds in each vaccinated flock. In countries where poultry are kept mainly in backyards and which are still developing their veterinary capacity, the minimum basic requirement is surveillance capable of detecting any antigenic variants that emerge [15].

Additional control measures to prevent virus spread (biosecurity, restrictions) could be enforced in the vaccination area, and guidelines for adequate management of disease outbreaks must be prepared and tested. Furthermore, under certain conditions, it might be useful to monitor the prevalence of infectious agents capable of producing immune suppression (e.g. infectious bursal disease, infectious anaemia and Marek's disease in chickens, and haemorrhagic enteritis in turkeys) and to implement specific vaccination programmes for their control.

Information system

The information system used to monitor the outcome of a vaccination programme should be adapted to the local situation. A minimum set of data should be collected and analysed to guarantee continuous monitoring of activities. Basic data on the vaccinated poultry population and the level of protection induced in target species and against possible circulation of avian influenza viruses should be available to veterinary authorities for decision-making. The information should fit the needs of decision-makers and should be used to plan and evaluate field operations.

Exit strategy

Vaccination of poultry against avian influenza is probably unsustainable in the long term because it is labour-intensive and very expensive; therefore, the conditions to be satisfied before a vaccination campaign is suspended must be defined. A feasible exit strategy should be developed from the beginning. The data collection system should provide information for identifying the main risk factors for disease introduction and spread in the area, for developing and applying adequate risk reduction measures and for identifying the conditions under which the vaccination plan could be reviewed or suspended.

Conclusions

Infection with high-pathogenicity viruses and with low-pathogenicity viruses capable of mutating into highly pathogenic forms can be controlled at source by risk reduction interventions, which include improved biosecurity, stamping-out, restrictions and vaccination. Use of avian influenza vaccines in poultry under different conditions must take into account the characteristics of the poultry-producing sector, the eco-epidemiological situation, the capacity of the veterinary infrastructure and the availability of adequate resources.

In rural areas where poultry are reared as a source of livelihood, immunization ensures food security and increases the sustainability of small-scale economies. Although poultry vaccination is a well-established practice for large farms and flocks, it is not always properly implemented at regional, area or compartment level, depending on the preparedness and capacity of the veterinary infrastructure and the level of cooperation between poultry farmers and other stakeholders. Education and awareness campaigns for rural communities in developing countries are essential parts of any intervention strategy, to increase participation and the effectiveness of avian influenza control programmes.

Countries should implement their avian influenza vaccination programmes only after they have adapted them to local conditions, to ensure efficacy and increase sustainability. Farsighted adaptation to local conditions is particularly important because, although human resources can be mobilized on the basis of personal responsibility and motivation to compensate for potential shortcomings in organization in the initial emergency phase, long-term sustainability requires more careful allocation of resources, bearing in mind that biosecurity is the bottom line of any exit strategy.

References

1 Capua I, Marangon S: Control of avian influenza in poultry. Emerg Infect Dis 2006;12:1319-1324.

2 Tian G, Zhang S, Li Y, Bu Z, Liu P, Zhou J, Li C, Shi J, Yu K, Chen H: Protective efficacy in chickens, geese and ducks of an H5N1-inactivated vaccine developed by reverse genetics. Virology 2005;341:153-162.

3 Qiao C, Tian G, Jiang Y, Li Y, Shi J, Yu K, Chen H (2006) Vaccines developed for H5 highly pathogenic avian influenza in China. Ann New York Acad Sci 2006;1081:182-191.

4 Tumpey TM, Kapczynsky DR, Swayne DE: Comparative susceptibility of chickens and turkeys to avian influenza A H7N2 virus infection and protective efficacy of a commercial avian influenza H7N2 virus vaccine. Avian Dis 2004;48:167-176.

5 van der Goot JA, Koch G, de Jong MC, van Boven M: Quantification of the effect of vaccination on transmission of avian influenza (H7N7) in chickens. Proc Nat Acad Sci USA 2005; 102:18141-18146.

6 Middleton D, Bingham J, Selleck P, Lowther S, Gleeson L, Lehrbach P, Robinson S, Rodenberg J, Kumar M, Andrew M: Efficacy of inactivated vaccines against H5N1 avian influenza infection in ducks. Virology 2007;359:66-71.

7 Marangon S, Busani L, Capua I: Practicalities of the implementation of a vaccination campaign for avian influenza. Avian Dis 2007;51(Suppl 1):297-303.

8 Ellis TM, Bousfield RB, Bissett LA, Dyrting KC, Luk GS, Tsim ST, Sturm-Ramirez K, Webster RG, Guan Y, Malik Peiris JS: Investigation of outbreaks of highly pathogenic H5N1 avian influenza in waterfowl and wild birds in Hong Kong in late 2002. Avian Pathol 2004; 33:492-505.

9 Chen H, Smith GJ, Li KS, Wang J, Fan XH, Rayner JM, Vijaykrishna D, Zhang JX, Zhang LJ, Guo CT, Cheung CL, Xu KM, Duan L, Huang K, Qinm K, Leung YH, Wu WL, Lu HR, Chen Y, Xia NS, Naipospos TS, Yuen KY, Hassan SS, Bahri S, Nguyen TD, Webster RG, Peiris JS, Guan Y (2006) Establishment of multiple sublineages of H5N1 influenza virus in Asia: implications for pandemic control. Proc Nat Acad Sci USA 2006;103:2845-2850.

10 FAO: FAO Position Paper on Recommendation on Prevention, Control and Eradication of Highly Pathogenica Avian Influenza in Asia. Rome, Food and Agriculture Organization of the United Nations, 2004. Available at:
http://www.fao.org/AG/AGAINFO/SUBJECTS/en/health/diseasescards/avian_fao.html.

11 FAO, OIM: A Global Strategy for the Progressive Control of Highly Pathogenic Avian Influenza (HPAI). Rome, Food and Agriculture Organization of the United Nations, and Paris, World Organization for Animal Health, 2005. Available at:
http://www.fao.org/ag/againfo/subjects/documents/ai/HPAIGlobalStrategy31Oct05.pdf.

12 Songserm T, Jam-on R, Sae-Heng N, Meemak N, Hulse-Post DJ, Sturm-Ramirez KM, Webster RG: Domestic ducks and H5N1 influenza epidemic, Thailand. Emerg Infect Dis 2006;12:575-581.

13 Swayne D: Principles for vaccine protection in chickens and domestic waterfowl against avian influenza. Ann NY Acad Sci 2006;1081:174-181.

14 Webster RG, Webby RJ, Hoffman E, Rodenberg J, Kumar M, Chu HJ, Seiler P, Krauss S, Songserm T: The imunogenicity and efficacy against H5N1 challenge of reverse genetics-derived H5N3 influenza vaccine in ducks and chickens. Virology 2006;351:303-311.

15 Sims LD: Lessons learned from Asian H5N1 outbreak control. Avian Dis 2007;51(Suppl 1):174-181.

Dr. Stefano Marangon, Istituto Zooprofilattico Sperimentale delle Venezie, Viale dell'Università 10, 35020, Legnaro (Padova), Italy.
E-mail: smarangon@izsvenezie.it

Dodet B and the Scientific & Technical Department of the OIE (eds): Vaccination: A Tool for the Control of Avian Influenza. Dev Biol (Basel). Basel, Karger, 2007, vol 130, pp 109-110.

Current Availability of Vaccines Including Vaccine Banks

P.G.H. Jones

International Federation for Animal Health (IFAH), Brussels, Belgium

Summary: Avian influenza can be considered one of the greatest global challenges the animal health sector has ever had to face. It is primarily a disease of animals and must be effectively managed by the veterinary community. Infection of humans in contact with the H5N1 virus continues to occur, however, with the possibility of mutations or re-assortment and the ever-present threat of the emergence of a pandemic. Therefore, whatever measures can be taken when outbreaks of avian influenza occur to reduce the amount of virus in circulation and potential human exposure must be reviewed constantly.
Conventional methods for controlling diseases of epizootic proportions, such as avian influenza, have tended to rely on bio-security and culling (stamping out) of enormous numbers of animals. Such approaches might not be adequate in areas of intensive animal husbandry, and society is questioning more and more the ethics of slaughtering millions of animals. The costs and economic impact of this strategy also has a considerable effect on the economy of the country or region in which the disease outbreak occurs.

Available Vaccines

Vaccination is an additional tool in the prevention and control of avian influenza in poultry. We describe here the vaccines that are available and their characteristics, while recognizing that vaccination alone cannot replace the other control measures of culling and stamping out. Avian influenza vaccines fall into two broad categories: conventional and recombinant.

Conventional

The conventional category includes both homologous and heterologous inactivated vaccines. The former have been used successfully but have the disadvantage that the virus is identical to that of the field infection, so that vaccinated birds cannot be differentiated from field-infected birds by serology. The manufacture of inactivated heterologous vaccines is similar to that of homologous ones, but, whereas the haemaglutinin is of the same type as that of the field virus, thereby stimulating active immunity, the neuramidase portion is different, resulting in alternative antibodies, which can be used to differentiate vaccinated from infected birds.

One of the main issues for consideration by authorities faced with the decision of whether to vaccinate is the impact on trade and exports of poultry meat and eggs from the country concerned. To provide the necessary assurance about the disease status of vaccinated birds, it is important to be able to differentiate infected from vaccinated animals (DIVA). This depends on the availability of appropriate diagnostic tests. Some are available, but their reliability and usefulness is a matter of debate and conjecture.

Recombinant

The number of recombinant vaccines is increasing, and both vector vaccines and those based on reverse genetics are available. The significant benefits of such advanced technology, particularly in respect of mass immunization techniques, is discussed, as are the advantages of the possibility of 'customizing' an influenza vaccine by assembling components of different viruses into a single vaccine virus.

A critical consideration for any vaccination campaign is the effectiveness of the available vaccines in preventing infection and, importantly, in preventing and stopping the shedding of virus from birds that are already infected. The available evidence appears to suggest that vaccinated birds excrete challenge virus for a shorter time and at a lower concentration than unvaccinated birds.

Vaccine banks

The concept of vaccine banks is usually considered in the context of emergency provision of vaccines against foot-and-mouth disease by dedicated laboratories established by the pharmaceutical companies concerned. In these special facilities, production is continuous, to meet the demands from countries around the world where the disease is endemic. The situation is different for avian influenza, for which vaccines are often manufactured at sites where other avian vaccines are also produced in large volumes. They therefore must compete for the finite capacity of the production facilities.

Consideration must therefore be given to the logistics of building up banks of vaccine that often have a biological shelf-life of only 1 year, while the manufacturing cycle can take up to 6 months and the predictability of requirements is often uncertain. Manufacturers must also decide which haemaglutinin and which neuramidase to select for vaccine manufacture, as well as the diagnostic tests available to implement a DIVA strategy, so that authorities are assured that they will be able to distinguish vaccinated from infected birds for trade purposes.

Dr. Peter Jones, International Federation for Animal Health (IFAM) 1, rue Defacaz B-1000, Brussels, Belgium
E-mail: p.jones@ifahsec.org

Dodet B and the Scientific & Technical Department of the OIE (eds): Vaccination: A Tool for the Control of Avian Influenza. Dev Biol (Basel). Basel, Karger, 2007, vol 130, pp 111-118.

Vaccination: a Means for Preserving Poultry Genetic Resources?

I. Hoffmann

Animal Production Service, Animal Production and Health Division, Food and Agricultural Organization of the United Nations, Rome, Italy

Keywords: poultry, genetic diversity, avian influenza (HPAI)

Summary: The genetic diversity of poultry worldwide is under threat. About 30% of reported poultry breeds were at risk of extinction before the crisis of highly pathogenic avian influenza (HPAI). Precise national statistics on the numbers of poultry producers, stocks, volume of production and the relative contributions of commercial and local stocks to production in developing countries are lacking. Although HPAI outbreaks have been occurring in East and South-East Asia for a number of years, many countries are still not sufficiently prepared to control outbreaks, and no contingency plans or information on spatial production include data on poultry genetic diversity. Comprehensive programmes for preventing HPAI disease should take into account the conservation of genetic diversity, which may include isolation or targeted protection of valuable stocks, through, for instance, vaccination and precautionary cryo-conservation of genetic material or other measures to ensure that genetic material can be spared from generalized culling measures in an outbreak. First, it will be necessary to characterize poultry genetic resources, and then to build inventories, including spatial information on breeds and valuable breeding stocks. Countries with low capacity to conduct vaccination campaigns often also have limited capacity to characterize or make inventories of genetic resources. Therefore, capacity- and institution-building are required in the animal production and health sector to ensure effective genetic stock assessment and successful vaccination programmes to preserve poultry genetic diversity in the event of disease introduction.

The Problem

Poultry keepers in developing countries are used to high losses, mainly due to predators, infectious diseases (e.g. Newcastle disease and chicken plague) or parasites. Highly pathogenic avian influenza (HPAI) due to H5N1 virus, a zoonotic disease that might potentially give rise to a human influenza pandemic, has received much public attention. Disease control measures, such as culling, movement control and a ban on 'wet' markets, are applied to varying degrees. Both the disease itself and its control measures have raised awareness of a possible threat to poultry genetic diversity. This paper first describes the current status of poultry genetic diversity and then looks into the impact of HPAI on the genetic resources. It concludes with an assessment of the role that targeted vaccination could play in protecting valuable genetic resources in the event of disease outbreaks.

Status of Poultry Genetic Diversity

FAO has finalized a 'State of the World's Animal Genetic Resources', the first assessment of domestic animal diversity [1]. The global databank contained in the Domestic Animal Diversity Information System (DAD-IS) was updated during preparation of the assessment and now contains information from 182 countries on 35 species of birds and mammals. DAD-IS reports breed-related information on 16 avian species and one fertile interspecies crossing (duck × Muscovy duck), with 3505 country breed populations. Chicken breeds make up the majority (63%) of avian breeds in the world, followed by duck (11%), goose (9%) and turkey (5%) breeds. Pigeons and guinea-fowl make up 3% each, and all other avian species 6%.

Many recorded breed populations occur in more than one country. As they may have a common gene pool and can therefore be considered the same breed, they have been linked and defined as 'transboundary' breeds. A total of 1644 local poultry breeds have been recorded, with records of 85 regional transboundary breeds, mostly in Europe and the Caucasus, and 157 international transboundary breeds, 101 of which are chicken (16 turkey, 15 goose, 12 duck). Population data, a prerequisite for breed management and assessment of risk status, are missing for many breeds and are available for only 39% of avian breeds [1].

Poultry breeding and breeding capacity in developing countries

Globally, poultry consumption is projected to grow up to 2030 at 2.5% per annum, which is faster than for other meats, and poultry consumption in developing countries is projected to grow at 3.4% per annum [2]. Developments in breeding, feeding and housing of poultry have resulted in an unprecedented increase in production and productivity in the past 20 years. The global poultry sector can be divided into two sub-sectors: large-scale commercial farms, dominated by international, developed country-based, vertically integrated companies, and small-scale farms that provide up to 90% of poultry production in some least-developed countries. Industrial production systems now account for an estimated 67% of global poultry meat production and 50% of egg production [3]. A fast reproduction cycle, a high reproduction rate, low unit costs, economies of scale in research and appropriation, and control of the produce are driving factors in the commercial sector.

For analytical reasons, FAO has grouped poultry production into four sectors by unit size and investment in biosecurity: industrial production with integrated biosecurity (sector 1), commercial poultry production with high (sector 2) or low (sector 3) biosecurity, and village or backyard production (sector 4). These systems are defined in different ways in different countries, which affects how they can be categorized for HPAI control and makes them difficult to compare from country to country. The systems do not fully reflect differences between bio-exclusion, i.e. measures to prevent pathogen introduction, and bio-containment, i.e. measures to prevent the spread of pathogens [4].

Most commercial layer and broiler stocks were created from a restricted genetic base in the past century in Europe and North America. Chicken breeding, both for layer and broiler breeds, and turkey breeding, are largely done by a few transnational breeding companies, which market their products worldwide and dominate the world market for poultry genetics. The primary breeders own pure lines and 'great-grandparent' stock. Primary breeders may be integrated or vertically aligned with grandparent flock customers, and these again with parent stock flocks, hatcheries and commercial production units located around the world. This results in a global trade network for day-old poultry, with elaborate logistics and transport at each level. The current players are managing the 6000 great-grandparent hens theoretically needed to provide the global supply of 800 billion eggs and the 11 000 pedigree hens needed to produce the 60 million tonnes of poultry meat [5]. In general, detailed information about commercial poultry breeding operations is scarce and difficult to obtain.

Despite the large number of poultry and poultry breeds kept by smallholders in developing countries, country reports prepared for the 'State of the World's Animal Genetic Resources' indicated that few countries had capacity in poultry breeding. This is due mainly to the large differences in commercial and local poultry production. Developing countries therefore have little incentive or interest in building a national breeding industry, as it is easier for them to import grandparent and parent stock. As a consequence, only 18% of countries in which chickens are kept reported that breeding was a priority, and only 13% had structured chicken breeding activities, and even less for other avian species. The proportion of breeds for which there are breeding programmes is larger in Europe and the Caucasus than in other regions [1].

The proportion of international transboundary breeds differs by region (Fig. 1), depending on the number of breeds that had been developed in the region before commercialization of the sector began and the current degree of commercialization of the sector.

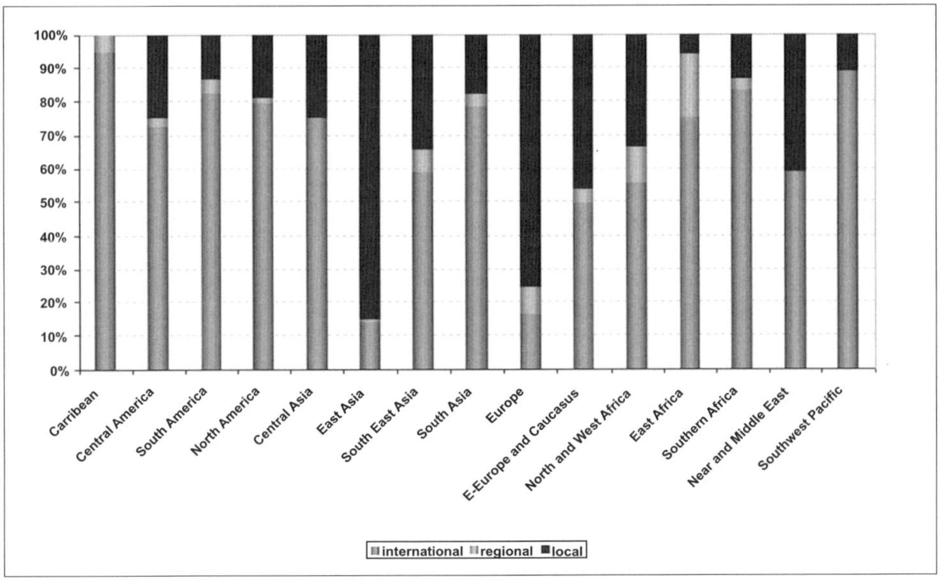

Fig. 1: Origin of chicken breeds, by subregion

Risk levels

The proportion of domesticated breeds classified as at risk is higher for avian (30%) than for mammalian species (16%). Of 2000 avian breeds, 524 are not at risk, and the risk status of 833 is unknown; 607 avian breeds are at risk, and 47 breeds, mainly chickens, are extinct. Some breeds of ducks, guinea-fowl and turkeys are also extinct [1] (Fig. 2). Globally, the avian species with the greatest number of breeds is chickens. The proportion of breeds at risk is high among chickens (33%), turkeys (34%) and geese (31%). The regions with the highest proportions of avian breeds classified as at risk are North America (79%) and Europe and the Caucasus (49%). These are the regions with the most highly specialized livestock industries, in which production is dominated by a small number of breeds and lines. In other regions, the risk status of most avian breeds is unknown (Fig. 2), and the assessment remains unsatisfactory.

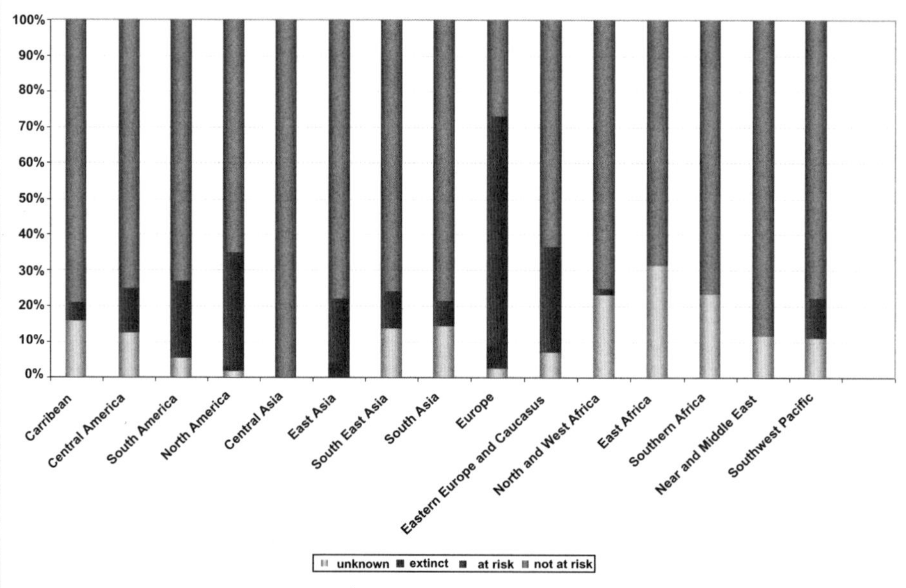

Fig. 2: Risk status of chicken breeds, by subregion

Impact of Highly Pathogenic Avian Influenza on Poultry Genetic Resources

Precise national statistics on the numbers of poultry producers, stocks and production and of the contribution of commercial and local stocks to production in developing countries are lacking. Although HPAI outbreaks have occurred in East and South-East Asia over the past few years, in most countries, none of the contingency plans or information on spatial production include poultry genetic diversity. Only in Hong Kong were valuable breeding poultry of rare Chinese breeds protected from culling. During the culls conducted in the first wave of disease control (2004), the genetic background of the culled birds was not recorded, and systematic data about which of the culled birds were infected and uninfected are missing.

We therefore have no hard data on the numbers or proportions of breeds affected by HPAI; only indirect assessments of the genetic background can be conducted. We can, with some certainty, exclude local breeds of chickens from sectors 1 and 2, but we cannot state with certainty that chickens in sector 4 are local breeds, owing to the long history of cross-breeding (e.g., operation coq raceur in Africa) and indiscriminate cross-breeding with exotics around centres of intensive poultry production in most countries. Countries without a significant commercial sector can be expected to have mainly local breeds in sector 4 and often also in sector 3.

In order to determine the impact of HPAI and HPAI control measures, the direct and indirect impacts must be distinguished. One weakness is differences in surveillance, reporting and communication in the four sectors [6]. Assessment of the direct impact of HPAI and HPAI control measures has provided no clear results. Country studies have shown higher incidences of HPAI in sectors 2 and 3 than in sectors 1 and 4 [7], and better physical biosecurity in sector 1 leads to reduced contact between the virus (and its carriers) and the host, whereas sector 4 does not play a substantial part in the market and transmission pathways.

Although there is anecdotal evidence that large-scale producers deliberately delay or avoid culling their stocks, direct disease control measures cannot be shown to discriminate against sector 4 farmers systematically. Nevertheless, culling policies affect large-scale and smallholders differently, and compensation policies in various countries have targeted them differently. There is anecdotal evidence that owners of backyard poultry have been excluded from official culling schemes, and therefore from compensation.

The picture of the potential indirect impact of HPAI control measures is clearer. Recently, it was proposed that the poultry sector should be restructured although few formal plans exist. This restructuring has the potential to marginalize smallholders and the local breeds they keep. The logic is to separate poultry units that are assumed to be biosecure (sectors 1 and 2) from those that are less biosecure (sectors 3 and 4). Programmes to increase biosecurity and to set up more integrated poultry chains designed for HPAI control have speeded up implementation of already existing government plans for relocation of large-scale production and market units in densely populated poultry areas into more remote areas (e.g. in Malaysia and Viet Nam). Closure or relocation of live poultry ('wet') markets, collection points and small slaughter points and subsequent exclusion of farmers in sectors 3 and 4 from the market chain might, however, have more negative implications for the future of local breeds than spatial relocation of the sectors. As the small-scale poultry sector makes a large contribution to production and direct marketing, market displacement will increase the risk for biodiversity [8]. In developed countries, the obligation to keep poultry indoors compromises the status of 'organic' or 'free-ranging' poultry [9]. Restructuring of the poultry sector could thus marginalize smallholders and add another risk for extinction of local breeds.

All disease control measures should take into account the complex relations between genetic diversity and disease ecology. The emergence of new avian influenza viruses and host shifts depend in part on the agro-ecological environment. In the case of HPAI, this environment is strongly affected by human activity, which changes the opportunities for host–virus contact, host density and species. Several studies have shown the complex effects on ecological relations of agricultural intensification and the related landscape alterations, changes in host species composition and density, increasing contacts between wild and domestic waterfowl and chickens, resulting in increasing virus pathogenicity and changing modes of disease transmission (from faecal or oral to respiratory) [10-12].

Studies of wild animals indicate that pathogens specialize for a common host [13,14]. The host habitat can be narrowed by, for example, intensification of animal production. The contribution of population genetic diversity to virus transmission dynamics needs further investigation. Mathematical models have shown that genetic diversity in a population affects both the probability of the occurrence of epidemics and their outcome. The lower the genetic diversity of a population, the greater the probability of extreme outcomes - either a completely healthy population or catastrophic epidemics. When the number of genotypes in a population increases, disease-dependent mortality during major epidemics decreases. Hence, standard epidemiological relations break down with heterogeneity, be it genetic, behavioural or environmental [15]. In commercial practice, reduced genetic diversity and increased unit size tend to go together: a large-scale commercial operation with a single source of genetic material is less heterogeneous than a multi-species multi-breed village flock.

Evidence from HPAI outbreaks indicates an important role for contact, density and trade (live poultry, products) in HPAI transmission. The effectiveness of bio-containment measures in parent stock operations, and particularly in hatcheries, is as yet unknown, and their role in disease transmission should be investigated. Although hard data are not yet available, recognition of the complex relations between disease ecology and genetics has resulted in reconsideration of the previous view that sector 1 is the most biosecure and sector 4 the least: pathogens can enter units with strong physical bio-exclusion measures [16]. It can be assumed, however, that great-grandparent operations present a low risk for spread of HPAI because of the high standards of health and biosecurity. In all situations, the biosecurity of the sectors and potential disease management measures should be based on case-by-case risk assessments.

Role of Vaccination

Vaccination against HPAI can help to protect valuable genetic stock (commercial, local, fancy) from disease and mortality and could spare them from culling in the case of a disease outbreak in the vicinity, as long as the policy takes this into account. The most important problem is the lack of information about the poultry sector described above and the fact that countries with little information about their poultry genetic resources usually also lack strong veterinary services. The management and protection of valuable genetic resources require breed characterization and registration, recording of population data and building of inventories, including spatial information, of breeds and valuable breeding stock in a country. The inventory should include a comprehensive risk assessment of all poultry subsectors.

As a second step, disease preparedness and emergency plans must be designed to address genetic resources, including emergency and preventive vaccination. This may involve isolation of valuable stocks and should also include precautionary cryo-conservation of genetic material or other measures to ensure that genetic material can be conserved in the case of an outbreak if birds have to be culled. The role of the private gene banks held by primary breeders and the public gene banks remains to be defined; gene banks should be established for local breeds and back-ups for commercial lines. Stored material is also useful for restocking if there is wide-scale culling, so that birds of the same genetic background are available.

Emergency ring or targeted vaccination should be undertaken to spare valuable stocks from culling. If valuable stocks in high-risk locations are vaccinated preventively, the vaccinated flocks should be registered so that they will be excluded from culling operations if they are not infected. Such stocks include commercial breeding stocks (great-grandparent and grandparent) and rare local breeds. High-risk locations would be identified in the risk assessment mentioned above and could include areas with a high probability of contact between domestic terrestrial poultry and domestic and wild waterfowl, or hatcheries in sectors 2 and 3 with low biosecurity.

Conclusions

Most national governments have only limited knowledge about their poultry sector, due to a 'closed' industry on the one hand and to the complex structure of the backyard sector on the other. Therefore, most countries seriously lack knowledge about most aspects of poultry genetic resources, while at the same time 30% of recognized poultry breeds were already under threat before the HPAI crisis. Characterization, inventories, spatial information and precautionary cryo-conservation of valuable material are necessary for management of poultry genetic resources, especially when under threat from HPAI. These measures should be developed in many countries for better management of the sector.

In view of the paucity of data on H5N1 HPAI virus and poultry genetic diversity, disease ecology, interaction of the virus with host genes and the wider host habitat, many research questions remain. These include the impact of vaccination on the diverse poultry species and breeds and the interaction between genetic resources, the structure of the poultry sector and HPAI occurrence. Poultry sector categories should be better defined and the overlap between breeds and poultry production sectors better identified in order to plan targeted interventions that take into account poultry genetic resources. Further research is needed in the complex area of disease ecology and genetic resources and to assess the probabilities of transmission to and between domestic flocks, including the design of dynamic models of disease transmission. The genetically controlled response of the host to infection also needs to be defined: genotyping of birds sampled from outbreaks and the creation and management of a database for genomic, phenotypic and epidemiological data would be crucial.

Genetic resources must be considered in risk assessments and in disease preparedness and contingency planning. Strategically used vaccination could be used to protect valuable genetic resources from HPAI and HPAI control measures. Many countries with poor capacity to conduct vaccination campaigns, however, also have a poor capacity to characterize genetic resources or to make an inventory.

Capacity- and institution-building in the animal production and health sector is a prerequisite for successful vaccination programmes, including those for conserving poultry genetic diversity.

Acknowledgements

I am grateful to Anni McLeod, Karin Schwabenbauer and Stephane de la Rocque for their comments on the manuscript and to Mateusz Wieczorek for preparing the charts from DAD-IS.

References

1 FAO: The State of the World's Animal Genetic Resources for Food and Agriculture, Rischkowsky B, Pilling, D (eds), Rome, Food and Agricultural Organization of the United Nations, 2007.

2 FAO: World Agriculture: Towards 2030/2050. Interim Report. Rome, Food and Agricultural Organization of the United Nations, 2006.

3 FAO: Classification and Characterization of World Livestock Production Systems. Update of the 1994 Livestock Production Systems Dataset with Recent Data. Groenewold J (ed) Unpublished report. Rome, Food and Agricultural Organization of the United Nations, 2004.

4 Otte J, Roland-Holst D, Pfeiffer D, Soares-Magalhaes R, Ruston J, Graham J, Silbergeld E: Industrial Livestock Production and Global Health Risks (Pro-poor Livestock Policy Initiative). Rome, Food and Agricultural Organization of the United Nations, 2007. http://www.fao.org/ag/againfo/projects/en/pplpi/docarc/rep-hpai_industrialisationrisks.pdf.

5 Preisinger R: Entwicklung, Stand und Perspektiven der Geflügelproduktion. Züchtungskunde 2005; 77:502-507.

6 Alders RG, Bagnol B: Effective communication: the key to efficient HPAI prevention and control. Worlds Poult Sci J 2007;63:139-147.

7 Rushton J, Viscarra R, Guerne-Bleich E, McLeod A: Impact of avian influenza outbreaks in the poultry sector of five South East Asian countries (Cambodia, Indonesia, Lao PDR, Thailand, Viet Nam): outbreak costs, responses and potential long term control. Worlds Poult Sci J 2005; 61:491-514.

8 Otte J, Roland-Holst D, Pfeiffer D (2006a) HPAI Control Measures and Household Incomes in Viet Nam (Pro-poor Livestock Policy Initiative). Rome, Food and Agricultural Organization of the United Nations, 2006. http://www.fao.org/ag/againfo/subjects/en/economics/facts/Vietnam-HPAI_DRH.pdf.

9 European Commission: Vaccination of Poultry against Highly Pathogenic Avian Influenza H5N1 (DIVA Strategy) (Discussion Paper SANCO/10103/2006 rev. 3), Brussels, 2006.

10 Chen H, Smith GJD, Li KS, Wang J, Fan XH, Rayner JM, Vijaykrishna D, Zhang JX, Zhang LJ, Guo CT, Cheung CL, Xu KM, Duan L, Huang K, Qin K, Leung YHC, Wu WL, Lu HR, Chen Y, Xia NS, Naipospos TSP, Yuen KY, Hassan SS, Bahri S, Nguyen TD, Webster RG, Peiris JSM, Guan Y: Establishment of multiple sublineages of H5N1 influenza virus in Asia: implications for pandemic control. Proc Natl Acad Sci USA 2006;103:2845-2850.

11 Webster RG, Peiris M, Chen H, Guan Y: H5N1 Outbreaks and enzootic influenza. Emerg Infect Dis 2006;12: 3–8. http://www.cdc.gov/ncidod/EID/vol12no01/pdfs/05-1024.pdf.

12 Gilbert M, Xiao X, Chaitaweesub P, Kalpravidh W, Premashthira S, Boles S, Slingenbergh J: Avian influenza, domestic ducks and rice agriculture in Thailand. Agric Ecosyst Environ 2007;119:409-415.

13 Little TJ: The evolutionary significance of parasitism: do parasite-driven genetic dynamics occur *ex silico*? J Evol Biol 2002;15:1-9.

14 Altizer S, Harvell D, Friedle E: Rapid evolutionary dynamics and disease threats to biodiversity. Trends Ecol Evolution Biol 2003;18:589-596.

15 Springbett AJ, MacKenzie K, Woolliams JA, Bishop SC: The contribution of genetic diversity to the spread of infectious diseases in livestock populations. Genetics 2003;165:1465-1474.

16 Otte J, Pfeiffer D, Tiensin T, Price L, Silbergeld E: Evidence-based Policy for Controlling HPAI in Poultry: Bio-security Revisited (Pro-poor Livestock Policy Initiative). Rome, Food and Agricultural Organization of the United Nations, 2006. http://www.fao.org/ag/againfo/projects/en/pplpi/docarc/rep-hpai_biosecurity.pdf.

Dr. Irene Hoffmann, Chief, Animal Production Service, Animal Production and Health Division, FAO, Viale delle Terme di Caracalla, 00153 Rome, Italy
E-mail: Irene.Hoffmann@fao.org

Dodet B and the Scientific & Technical Department of the OIE (eds): Vaccination: A Tool for the Control of Avian Influenza. Dev Biol (Basel). Basel, Karger, 2007, vol 130, p 119.

SESSION V

Vaccines and Research

Chairperson: *J. Lubroth*, FAO, Italy

Dodet B and the Scientific & Technical Department of the OIE (eds): Vaccination: A Tool for the Control of Avian Influenza. Dev Biol (Basel). Basel, Karger, 2007, vol 130, pp 121-131.

Current Developments in Avian Influenza Vaccines, including Safety of Vaccinated Birds as Food

D.E. Swayne, D.L. Suarez

Southeast Poultry Research Laboratory, Agricultural Research Service, Department of Agriculture, Athens, Georgia, United States of America

Keywords: vaccine, avian influenza, DIVA, HPAI, safety

Summary: Until recently, most vaccines against avian influenza were based on oil-emulsified inactivated low- or high-pathogenicity viruses. Now, recombinant fowl pox and avian paramyxovirus type 1 vaccines with avian influenza H5 gene inserts (+ or – N1 gene insert) are available and licensed. New technologies might overcome existing limitations to make available vaccines that can be grown in tissue culture systems for more rapid production; provide optimized protection, as a result of closer genetic relations to field viruses; allow mass administration by aerosol, in drinking-water or *in ovo*; and allow easier strategies for identifying infected birds within vaccinated populations (DIVA). The technologies include avian influenza viruses with partial gene deletions, avian influenza–Newcastle disease virus chimeras, vectored vaccines such as adenoviruses and Marek's disease virus, and subunit vaccines. These new methods should be licensed only after their purity, safety, efficacy and potency against avian influenza viruses have been demonstrated, and, for live vectored vaccines, restriction of viral transmission to unvaccinated birds. Use of vaccines in countries affected by highly pathogenic avian influenza will not only protect poultry but will provide additional safety for consumers. Experimental studies have shown that birds vaccinated against avian influenza have no virus in meat and minimal amounts in eggs after HPAI virus challenge, and that replication and shedding from their respiratory and alimentary tracts is greatly reduced.

Introduction

Protection elicited by infection with avian influenza virus or vaccination with vaccines against this virus results from a combination of humoral, cell-mediated and innate immunity. The humoral immune response in birds provides protection mainly by raising antibodies against haemagglutinin and, to a lesser extent, neuraminidase surface proteins, but antibodies against internal proteins have not been shown to be protective in birds [1]. The protection by haemagglutinin and neuraminidase is subtype-specific. The cell-mediated immune response, usually produced by infection with live avian influenza viruses and not with inactivated vaccines, has been shown to provide broad protection in experimental studies with multiple haemagglutinin subtypes of avian influenza viruses [2], but its contribution to immunity in field vaccination programmes is largely unknown. Innate immunity provides protection through macrophage, heterophil and other cells that secrete cytokines, which affect initiation or termination of avian influenza viral infection. This paper focuses on the humoral immune response. Several aspects of the avian immune system should be explored, including: the effect of heterosubtypic immunity against the M2 protein on protection of birds against all avian influenza viruses, similar to the heterosubtypic immunity against influenza A viruses in mouse models; the potential collective effect of immune responses against all avian influenza viral proteins in contrast to immunity to haemagglutinin alone in protecting against antigen drift; and enhancement of humoral, cell-mediated and innate immune responses with live virus vaccines and with inactivated vaccines.

Avian Influenza Vaccine Technology

Licensed avian influenza vaccines for use in the field and experimentally are based on four broad categories of technique [3]: inactivated whole avian influenza virus, haemagglutinin expressed in vitro and potentially other avian influenza viral proteins, haemagglutinin expressed in vivo and potentially other avian influenza viral proteins, and naked nucleic acids. The inactivated vaccines are mainly based on low-pathogenicity avian influenza viruses from field outbreaks, occasionally highly pathogenic avian influenza (HPAI) viruses and, most recently, reverse genetic-produced strains based on the haemagglutinin and neuraminidase from a field avian influenza virus, usually by altering the HPAI virus haemagglutinin proteolytic cleavage site to low-pathogenicity virus haemagglutinin and the remaining virus genes from a high-growth influenza A vaccine virus [3,4]. The viruses are grown in embryonating chicken eggs, and the infected chorioallantoic fluid is collected, chemically inactivated and emulsified in mineral oil adjuvant. With the in-vitro expression systems, the immunogen (e.g. haemagglutinin) is produced in a laboratory or manufacturing plant in eukaryotic tissue cultures (plant and animal cells), plants, yeast, bacteria or viruses (vaccinia). An example of the latter system is a baculovirus (insect virus) vector that can grow in an insect cell culture and produce the immunogen. All the immunogenic protein is produced externally to the bird host. In contrast, in the in-vivo systems, the immunogen is produced within the bird host by use of a live bacterial or viral vector such as fowl poxvirus, adenovirus, avian leukosis virus, infectious laryngotracheitis virus, Newcastle disease virus, avian influenza-Newcastle disease chimeric virus, Marek's disease herpesvirus, *Salmonella* spp. or other organisms. The naked nucleic acids are avian influenza viral cDNA contained within various plasmids with mammalian promotors [5]. The DNA vaccines are not addressed in this paper because their current limitation is the large quantity of expensive nucleic acid needed to produce a protective immune response in chickens. DNA vaccines will be prohibitively expensive for use in the field until new promotors are found to reduce the number of vaccinations and the quantity of nucleic acids used.

Goals of Avian Influenza Vaccines and Vaccination

When properly used, avian influenza vaccines will protect birds by increasing their resistance to infection, preventing clinical signs and death, reducing the shedding of field virus when the birds become infected, preventing contact transmission, providing long protection from both low and high exposures and protecting against a changing virus. With the antigenic drift in field avian influenza viruses, however, vaccine strains have a finite lifespan, although they have a longer effective life than human influenza vaccine strains [3,4].

Avian influenza vaccines are not a complete solution, however, but only one part of a comprehensive control strategy, because vaccinated flocks can have 'silent' infections, e.g. virus shedding without clinical signs, and they should be monitored to assess the effectiveness of vaccination and other control components by special virological and serological surveillance procedures. In order that the next generation of vaccines and vaccine use is effective, the latest science must be used to address the following issues:

- the need for mass vaccination methods, such as administration in water, feed, spray and *in ovo*;
- increasing use of biotechnology to address antigenic drift and to increase the antigen content of inactivated avian influenza vaccines;
- viable vaccination protocols and combinations of vaccines for use in the field; for example, effective use of virus-vectored vaccines might depend on knowledge of the virus and vector maternal antibody levels in birds;
- improved adjuvants for inactivated avian influenza vaccines to elicit a better immune response in waterfowl;
- vaccines and vaccination protocols that result in longer, enhanced immunity with few vaccinations; and
- consistent quality of inactivated avian influenza vaccines, such that an adequate amount of antigen for the type of adjuvant is included and the vaccines meet international standards for purity, safety, efficacy and potency.

Mass Vaccination

Until recently, all avian influenza vaccines were administered by handling and injecting each bird, and most of the vaccines were inactivated viruses in an oil adjuvant base. Since 1998, live recombinant fowl poxvirus vaccines with an avian influenza H5 gene insert have been used in Central America. Both types of vaccine require parenteral administration, but experimental and field data indicate that they are efficacious. Administration of these vaccines is labour-intensive, and birds become stressed during handling; furthermore, the vaccines are relatively expensive and are used mainly for high-value birds and in countries with abundant low-cost labour. Future vaccines must be designed that allow mass vaccination, such as in water, feed or *in ovo*, or by spray application, so that they can be used for low-cost meat production poultry.

Topical application

Initial studies have shown limited protection when inactivated avian influenza vaccine or recombinant fowl poxvirus vector vaccine is given topically, intranasally, intratracheally or into the conjunctival sac (i.e. by eye drop). A human replication-deficient adenovirus-vectored vaccine with an H5 gene insert (A/Vietnam/1203/04 (H5N1) was tested for efficacy in 3-week-old white Leghorn chickens after subcutaneous and intranasal administration of $10^{10.6}$ virus particles per chicken [6]. Three weeks later, the chickens were challenged with 10^6 mean chicken embryo infectious doses (EID_{50}) of the HPAI virus strain. The subcutaneously vaccinated chickens were completely protected from illness and death, while 50% of the intranasally vaccinated chickens and 100% of those that received the vector alone became ill and died (Table 1). In the subcutaneously vaccinated chickens, field virus shedding from the alimentary and respiratory tracts was significantly reduced, by over 10^3 EID_{50}. Although this adenovirus-vectored vaccine conferred protection after subcutaneous injection, mass application to the respiratory tract would not result in protection.

Table 1: Adenovirus-vectored vaccine with H5 gene insert ($10^{10.6}$ virus particles) given subcutaneously or intranasally to 3-week-old white Leghorn chickens challenged at 6 weeks of age with A/Vietnam/1203/04 (H5N1) HPAI virus

d-Adenovirus vaccine	Morbidity	Mortality (time to death in days)	Virus isolation 2 days after challenge ($\log_{10}$ EID_{50} titre/ml)	
			Oral swab	Cloacal swab
Vector (subcutaneous)	10/10	10/10 (1.8)	10/10 (6.96)	10/10 (6.26)
Avian influenza virus H5 (subcutaneous)	0/10	0/10	9/10 (3.84)	0/10 (<0.9)
Vector (intranasal)	10/10	10/10 (1.8)	ND	ND
Avian influenza virus H5 (intranasal)	05/10	10/10 (6.0)	ND	ND

ND, not done
The numbers of sick and dead birds were reported for the total group, and the mean time to death was calculated. At 2 days after challenge, virus shedding was assayed in the respiratory (oropharyngeal swab) and alimentary (cloacal swab) tracts [6].

Fowl pox is a disease of chickens transmitted by contact with abraded skin, but it can also be transmitted by inhalation, resulting in tracheal pox lesions, or ‘wet pox’. Fowl pox vaccines, including the recombinant fowl poxvirus-avian influenza virus vaccine, must be injected parenterally to elicit a consistent protective immune response, as topical application (intranasal, intratracheal or conjunctival sac) of fowl pox vaccines is not effective. The recombinant fowl poxvirus-avian influenza H5 virus vaccine has some advantages over inactivated vaccines as it can be administered in the hatchery and raises earlier immunity than inactivated vaccines. Furthermore, it is used in biosecure hatcheries and not on farms, so the risk for spread of avian influenza virus by vaccination crews is eliminated.

A recombinant Newcastle disease virus vaccine vector system has been designed [7], which has advantages for mass application, because live Newcastle disease vaccines are already used in chicken and turkey production in most of the world and are easily applied by spray, and the recombinant vaccines provide protection against Newcastle disease, another exotic viral disease common in much of the developing world. Initial studies in 2003 demonstrated that use of recombinant Newcastle disease virus-avian influenza H7 virus vaccine protected birds against Newcastle disease and H7 HPAI viruses [8]. Subsequently, several laboratories have demonstrated that recombinant Newcastle disease virus containing an avian influenza haemagglutinin gene insert can protect chickens from challenge with both Newcastle disease virus and HPAI virus:

- Recombinant Newcastle disease virus-avian influenza H7 virus (A/chicken/New York/13142-5/94 (H7N2)) administered in eye drops ($10^{5.7-6.1}$ EID_{50}) to chickens at 2 and 4 weeks of age protected 90-100% of birds from illness and death after intranasal challenge at 6 weeks of age with 10^5 EID_{50} of the Fontana/73 strain of velogenic viserotropic Newcastle disease virus and A/Steele/59 (H7N7) HPAI virus [9].
- Oculonasal administration of 10^6 EID_{50} recombinant Newcastle disease virus-avian influenza H5 virus (A/Bar-headed Goose/Qinghai/05 (H5N1)) vaccine to 1-week-old chickens protected the birds from 10^3 mean chicken lethal doses (CLD_{50}) of the F48E9 strain of velogenic viserotropic Newcastle disease virus or 10^3 CLD_{50} of HPAI virus strains A/Goose/Guangdong/96 (H5N1) and A/Bar-headed Goose/Qinghai/05 (H5N1) [10].
- Administration in eye drops of $10^{5.5}$ EID_{50} recombinant Newcastle disease virus-avian influenza H5 virus (strain not reported) to 10-day-old chickens protected 90% of the birds after combined intranasal and conjunctival sac challenge with 10^6 EID_{50} with A/chicken/Mexico/Querataro/95 (H5N2) HPAI virus at 31 days of age [11].
- Oculonasal administration of 10^6 EID_{50} recombinant Newcastle disease virus-avian influenza H5 virus (A/chicken/Italy/98 (H5N2)) to 3-week-old chickens provided 100% protection after challenge with $10^{7.7}$ EID_{50} of A/chicken/Italy/98 (H5N2) HPAI virus [12].

Two of these recombinant Newcastle disease virus-avian influenza H5 virus vaccines have been licensed for use in poultry in China and Mexico, respectively.

Another vaccine that could be given by mass vaccination is a genetically modified infectious laryngotracheitis vaccine virus with an H5 haemagglutinin gene insert from A/chicken/Italy/98 (H5N2) [13]. Vaccination of 18 week-old layers with 10^5 plaque-forming units of the vaccine provided 100% protected from intranasal challenge 4 weeks later with 10^8 EID_{50} of A/chicken/Italy/98 (H5N2) or A/chicken/Scotland/59 (H5N1) HPAI virus.

Other techniques show promise for mass immunizing vector systems for avian influenza:

- An avirulent double gene deletant *Salmonella* vector and similarly derived *Salmonella* vaccines are already licensed in the USA for protection against *Salmonella* and could be used to vector avian influenza genes [14].

- The avian influenza virus could be a vector as a result of point mutations in one or more genes or partial deletions of genes, which would reduce virulence, limit transmission and restrict replication, as has been done by cold adaptation of some human influenza A vaccine strains.
- An avian influenza virus-Newcastle disease virus chimera, in which a portion of the avian influenza virus neuraminidase gene is replaced by part of the Newcastle disease virus haemagglutinin-neuraminidase gene, protects against both Newcastle disease and avian influenza [9].

Administration *in ovo*

Many broiler chickens receive vaccines against Marek's disease and other diseases at 18 days of incubation (i.e. *in ovo*), saving labour and vaccine costs and eliciting an earlier immune response than vaccination after hatching. Development of avian influenza vaccines for administration *in ovo* would be advantageous for commercial broiler production. A preliminary study showed that manual administration of inactivated oil-emulsified avian influenza vaccine A/turkey/Wisconsin/68 *in ovo* provided protection from illness and death after high-dose challenge with A/chicken/Pennsylvania/1370/83 (H5N2)) HPAI virus [15]; however, additional research is needed to determine the compatibility or lack thereof of combined administration of inactivated avian influenza vaccine and live Marek's disease vaccine. Administration of adenovirus-vectored vaccine with an avian influenza H5 gene insert from A/turkey/Wisconsin/68 (H5N9) *in ovo* protected chickens from illness and death after challenge at 34 days of age with an HPAI virus (A/chicken/Queretaro/14588-19/95 (H5N2)) [16]. The vaccine also decreased the amount of HPAI virus shed on day 7 after challenge, but the reduction in virus shedding was not seen at earlier times. Vaccination *in ovo* with inactivated avian influenza vaccines might be feasible if the vaccine could be mixed and coadministered with live Marek's disease vaccine. Vectoring of avian influenza viral haemagglutinin in a Marek's disease virus might also result in an avian influenza vaccine that could be administered *in ovo*.

Biotechnology Solutions

Antigenic drift in haemagglutinin of avian influenza viruses

A major problem with human influenza vaccine is failure due to antigenic drift of the field viruses away from the vaccine strains, which necessitates changes in vaccine strains every 3-5 years. Avian influenza vaccine strains have been used for much longer; for example, a 1968 North American inactivated H5N2 vaccine strain and recombinant fowl pox with an H5 gene from a 1983 Irish HPAI virus both protected against a 2003 Republic of Korea H5N1 HPAI virus [3]. The report of a series of experiments. with a recombinant fowl pox-H5-Ire/83 vaccine showed excellent protection against morbidity and mortality in chickens challenged with various H5 HPAI viruses isolated between 1959 and 2005 (Table 2). There was, however, an inverse correlation between differences in the challenge virus-vaccine virus haemagglutinin sequence and the ability to reduce replication and shedding from the respiratory tract. Nevertheless, the reduction in replication was significant even when the haemagglutinin differences were as high as 13% [17].

Table 2: Protection of chickens from death by subcutaneous vaccination at 1 day of age with recombinant fowl pox-H5-Ire/83 and intranasal challenge at 3 weeks of age with 10^{5-6} EID_{50} of various HPAI viruses isolated between 1959 and 2005

Challenge virus	Subtype	Haemagglutinin similarity to vaccine (%)	Mortality
A/ck/Scotland/59	H5N1	92	0/10
A/tern/S. Africa/61	H5N3	93.1	0/10
A/tk/Ontario/66	H5N9	89.1	0/10
A/ck/PA/83	H5N2	87.3	0/10
A/tk/Ireland/83	H5N8	100	0/10
A/tk/England	H5N1	94.2	0/10
A/ck/Queretaro/95	H5N2	89.3	0/10
A/HK/156/97	H5N1	90.2	0/10
A/ck/S. Korea/03	H5N1	89.9	0/10
A/ck/Vietnam/04	H5N1	88.4 (estimated)	0/22
A/WS/Mongolia/05	H5N1	89.7	1/8
Control	–	–	80-100%

The challenge viruses had 87.3–100% haemagglutinin sequence similarity with avian influenza H5 in the vaccine strain. Compiled from [3,17] and unpublished data.

Although the data support broad cross-protection within the H5 subtype for HPAI viruses, new data suggest that there is limited cross-protection among H7 HPAI viruses [Unpublished data]. With recombinant fowl pox technology, a vaccine with an H7 gene insert from A/chicken/Victoria/1/85 (H7N7) protected chickens against A/chicken/Pakistan/1369-CR2/95 (H7N3) HPAI virus but not against A/turkey/Italy/4580/99 (H7N1). Furthermore, chickens vaccinated with other recombinant fowl pox vaccines were protected against A/turkey/Italy/4580/99 (H7N1) when the vaccine contained the homologous haemagglutinin gene insert but not if the vaccine had haemagglutinin inserts from A/chicken/Victoria/1/85 (H7N7) or A/turkey/Virginia/66/02 (H7N2). This indicates that there are sufficient differences between H7 viruses that broad cross-protection within the H7 subtype will not occur.

The idea that antigenic drift phenomena contribute to the failure of poultry avian influenza vaccine was clearly demonstrated with respect to Central American H5N2 low-pathogenicity avian influenza viruses [18]. The 1994 Mexican H5N2 avian influenza strain in inactivated vaccines was protective against the 1994 low-pathogenicity and HPAI viruses, but the same vaccine strain did not protect chickens from a 1998 Mexican H5N2 low-pathogenicity or a 2002 Guatemalan H5N2 low-pathogenicity virus. These results suggest that avian influenza vaccine strains should be tested regularly, such as biannually, against the current circulating field strains to assess their ability to protect. The testing should include both molecular sequence comparisons, antigen cross-protection in vitro and vaccine efficacy trials in vivo. In view of the endemicity of H5N1 HPAI viruses in Asia and continuing antigenic drift, the usefulness of H5 low-pathogenicity field viruses as vaccine strains will have a limited life span. Future vaccines must be derived by biotechnology, such as avian influenza virus reverse genetic clone technology, to produce more relevant low-pathogenicity strains for inactivated vaccine [19,20].

Can neuraminidase-based vaccines provide protection?

The possibility has been raised of designing and using avian influenza vaccines based on neuraminidase, either as a 'stand-alone' vaccine or as an adjunct to haemagglutinin-based vaccine. In a recent study, a recombinant fowl pox with an N1 gene insert from A/turkey/Italy/4580/99 (H7N1) did not protect chickens challenged with the same virus. In another study, however, vaccination of chicken with N2 neuraminidase in DNA, baculovirus-generated N2 or replication-deficient Venezuelan equine encephalitis with an N2 gene insert gave partial protection against N2 HPAI virus challenge; increasing the number of vaccinations increased antibody titres and improved protection [21]. Currently, neuraminidase-based vaccines are not being considered for use in poultry.

Practical considerations for vaccine use

Many viral vector techniques can be used to produce relevant avian influenza vaccines, including fowl poxvirus and Marek's disease virus. Live virus vectors have a huge advantage in that a replaceable cassette system can be used that allows the design and exchange of an insert for a closer match to emerging avian influenza field viruses. Developing a relevant vaccine is, however, only the first step. Additional knowledge is needed about use of the new vaccines in the field for generating optimal immunity. New vaccination protocols will be needed that provide:

- an understanding of the impact of maternal antibodies or pre-existing active immunity on replication of a vectored vaccine and of use of the vectored product to maximize immunity;
- information on the susceptibility of host species to the vectored vaccines; and
- vaccination protocols with optimal use of different combinations of vaccines to achieve acceptable immunity under field conditions.

Immunization to Prevent Highly Pathogenic Avian Influenza in Poultry Products

Avian influenza viral infections affect international trade in poultry and poultry products, especially in countries that have outbreaks of HPAI. H5N1 HPAI viruses have caused human infection with fatalities, but the primary risk factor for infection is direct or indirect exposure to infected poultry, especially sick or dead birds, and not consumption of poultry products [22-25]. Vaccination of poultry at risk is important in reducing human exposure by reducing the virus load in respiratory secretions, faeces and carcasses, thus eliminating the source of virus for human infections.

Systemic infection has been demonstrated in HPAI virus-infected chickens, and virus has been found in blood, bone and meat; but no low-pathogenicity virus has been found in these tissues from chickens infected with this virus [26]. Feeding of HPAI virus-infected meat transmitted the virus to naive chickens when the meat contained large quantities of the virus. In additional experiments, the H5N1 HPAI virus was found in meat from chickens, ducks, Japanese quail and geese that had been inoculated intranasally with various H5N1 HPAI viruses originating from birds (2003-2005) and humans (2004-2005). In the field, H5N1 HPAI virus has been isolated from raw frozen duck meat originating in China and imported to the Republic of Korea (2001) and Japan (2003) [27,28]. In experimental studies, H5N1 HPAI virus was not recovered from the meat of vaccinated chickens or domestic ducks after intranasal exposure to H5N1 HPAI viruses [26,29].

Less is known about contamination of eggs with avian influenza virus. In a recent study of 24 white Leghorn adult laying chickens, intranasal challenge with A/Pennsylvania/1/83 (H5N2) low-pathogenicity avian influenza virus produced a typical respiratory infection and a drop in egg production [Unpublished data]. No virus was recovered from the albumen or yolk of the eggs during the 14-day study, but very low levels were recovered from the eggshell surface on days 2 and 3 after challenge, presumably from contamination in the cloaca as a result of alimentary-tract infection. In contrast, intranasal inoculation of 24 white Leghorn adult laying chickens with A/chicken/Pennsylvania/1370/83 (H5N2) HPAI virus resulted in cessation of egg production by day 4 after challenge, and HPAI virus was recovered from the eggshell, albumen and yolks of 17 of 22 eggs laid on days 2 and 3 after challenge, but not from eggs laid on day 1 after challenge. All chickens had died or stopped laying by day 4 after challenge. This finding supports the results of previous studies showing that HPAI viruses cause systemic infection in chickens and result in localization of the virus in the internal contents of eggs laid during the 2 days before death. In an experimental study in 24 white Leghorn adult laying chickens, in which 12 birds were given sham vaccine (oil adjuvant and sterile chorioallantoic egg fluid) and 12 were vaccinated with an inactivated H5 avian influenza vaccine (oil emulsified A/Turkey/WI/68 (H5N9)), the number of HPAI-virus positive eggs laid after challenge with A/Pennsylvania/1370/83 (H5N2) HPAI virus was decreased from 39% to 16%, but the eggs from chickens vaccinated against avian influenza had less virus than eggs from the sham-vaccinated group.

Conclusions

Vaccines have been valuable in the control of avian influenza, which until recently were primarily inactivated avian influenza vaccines and recombinant fowl pox-avian influenza virus-H5 vaccine. Live vectors for mass vaccination will, however, result in better application methods because of the greater ease of application and the reduced cost. Nevertheless, vaccination protocols should be designed to optimize use, such as by overcoming maternal or existing active immunity and developing improved application methods, such as *in ovo* in the industrial sector.

Antigenic drift will continue to be a challenge for the efficacy of avian influenza vaccines, but current and emerging biotechnology, such as avian influenza reverse genetic cloning systems and replaceable cassettes in live vaccine vectors, will result in effective vaccines more rapidly. Immunization can prevent or reduce replication of HPAI virus in meat, eggs and viscera of poultry, adding a safety feature to avian influenza control.

Acknowledgements

The authors thank Matt Sylte, Joan Beck, James Doster, Kira Moresco and Susanne DeBlois of the Southeast Poultry Research Laboratory for technical assistance and Michel Bublot, Nikki Pritchard and Tom Mickle of Merial, Inc. for technical contributions to the data on recombinant fowl pox.

References

1 Swayne DE, Halvorson DA: Influenza. In: Saif YM, Glisson JR, Fadly AM, McDougald LR, Nolan L (eds) Diseases of Poultry. Ames, Iowa, Blackwell, 2008.

2 Seo SH, Webster RG: Cross-reactive, cell-mediated immunity and protection of chickens from lethal H5N1 influenza virus infection in Hong Kong poultry markets. J Virol 2001;75:2516-2525.

3 Swayne DE: Application of new vaccine technologies for the control of transboundary diseases. Dev Biol (Basel) 2004, 119:219-228.

4 Swayne DE: Principles for vaccine protection in chickens and domestic waterfowl against avian influenza: emphasis on Asian H5N1 high pathogenicity avian influenza. Ann NY Acad Sci 2006;1081:174-181.

5 Suarez DL, Schultz-Cherry S: The effect of eukaryotic expression vectors and adjuvants on DNA vaccines in chickens using an avian influenza model. Avian Dis 2000;44:861-868.

6 Gao W, Soloff AC, Lu X, Montecalvo A, Nguyen DC, Matsuoka Y, Robbins PD, Swayne DE, Donis RO, Katz JM, Barratt-Boyes SM, Gambotto A: Protection of mice and poultry from lethal H5N1 avian influenza virus through adenovirus-based immunization. J Virol 2006;80:1959-1964.

7 Nakaya T, Cros J, Park MS, Nakaya Y, Zheng HY, Sagrera A, Villar E, Garcia-Sastre A, Palese P: Recombinant Newcastle disease virus as a vaccine vector. J Virol 2001;75:11868-11873.

8 Swayne DE, Suarez DL, Schultz-Cherry S, Tumpey TM, King DJ, Nakaya T, Palese P, Garcia-Sastre A: Recombinant paramyxovirus type 1-avian influenza-H7 virus as a vaccine for protection of chickens against influenza and Newcastle disease. Avian Dis 2003;47:1047-1050.

9 Park M, Steel J, Garcia-Sastre A, Swayne D, Palese P: Engineered viral vaccine constructs with dual specificity: avian influenza and Newcastle disease. Proc Natl Acad Sci USA 2006;103:8203-8208.

10 Ge J, Deng G, Wen Z, Tian G, Wang Y, Shi J, Wang X, Li Y, Hu S, Jiang Y, Yang C, Yu K, Bu Z, Chen H: Newcastle disease virus-based live attenuated vaccine completely protects chickens and mice from lethal challenge of homologous and heterologous H5N1 avian influenza viruses. J Virol 2007;81:150-158.

11 Lozano B, Soto E, Sarfati D, Castro F, Gay M, Antillon A: A novel engineered live viral vaccine against Newcastle disease and avian influenza subtype H5. In: Book of abstracts. FAO/OIE Conference on Vaccination: A Tool for the Control of Avian Influenza, Verona, 2007. Rome, Food and Agricultural Organization of the United Nations, 2007.

12 Veits J, Wiesner D, Fuchs W, Hoffmann B, Granzow H, Starick E, Mundt E, Schirrmeier H, Mebatsion T, Mettenleiter TC, Romer-Oberdorfer A: Newcastle disease virus expressing H5 hemagglutinin gene protects chickens against Newcastle disease and avian influenza. Proc Natl Acad Sci USA 2006;103:8197-8202.

13 Luschow D, Werner O, Mettenleiter TC, Fuchs W: Protection of chickens from lethal avian influenza A virus infection by live-virus vaccination with infectious laryngotracheitis virus recombinants expressing the hemagglutinin (H5) gene. Vaccine 2001;19:4249-4259.

14 Cole K, Tayton SL, Cox MM, Kwon YM, Berghman WJ, Bottje WJ, Hargis BM: Development and primary evaluation of a recombinant salmonella expressing M2e and CD154 as a vaccine vector for avian influenza. In: Book of abstracts. FAO/OIE Conference on Vaccination: A Tool for the Control of Avian Influenza, Verona, 2007. Rome, Food and Agricultural Organization of the United Nations, 2007.

15 Stone H, Mitchell B, Brugh M: In ovo vaccination of chicken embryos with experimental Newcastle disease and avian influenza oil-emulsion vaccines. Avian Dis 1997; 41:856-863.

16 Toro H, Tang DC, Suarez DL, Sylte MJ, Pfeiffer J, Van Kampen KR: Protective avian influenza in ovo vaccination with non-replicating human adenovirus vector. Vaccine 2007;25:2886-2891.

17 Swayne DE, Garcia M, Beck JR, Kinney N, Suarez DL: Protection against diverse highly pathogenic avian influenza viruses in chickens immunized with a recombinant fowl pox vaccine containing an H5 avian influenza hemagglutinin gene insert. Vaccine 2000;18:1088-1095.

18 Lee CW, Senne DA, Suarez DL: Effect of vaccine use in the evolution of Mexican lineage H5N2 avian influenza virus. J Virol 2004;78:8372-8381.

19 Lee CW, Senne DA, Suarez DL: Generation of reassortant influenza vaccines by reverse genetics that allows utilization of a DIVA (Differentiating Infected from Vaccinated Animals) strategy for the control of avian influenza. Vaccine 2004;22:3175-3181.

20 Liu M, Wood JM, Ellis T, Krauss S, Seiler P, Johnson C, Hoffmann E, Humberd J, Hulse D, Zhang Y, Webster RG, Perez DR: Preparation of a standardized, efficacious agricultural H5N3 vaccine by reverse genetics. Virology 2003;314:580-590.

21 Sylte MJ, Hubby B, Suarez DL: Influenza neuraminidase antibodies provide partial protection for chickens against highly pathogenic avian influenza infection. Vaccine 2007;25:3763-3772.

22 Mounts AW, Kwong H, Izurieta HS, Ho Y, Au T, Lee M, Buxton BC, Williams SW, Mak KH, Katz JM, Thompson WW, Cox NJ, Fukuda K: Case–control study of risk factors for avian influenza A (H5N1) disease, Hong Kong, 1997. J Infect Dis 1999;180:505-508.

23 Bridges CB, Lim W, Hu-Primmer J, Sims L, Fukuda K, Mak KH, Rowe T, Thompson WW, Conn L, Lu X, Cox NJ, Katz JM: Risk of influenza A (H5N1) infection among poultry workers, Hong Kong, 1997-1998. J Infect Dis 2002;185:1005-1010.

24 Tran TH, Nguyen TL, Nguyen TD, Luong TS, Pham PM, Nguyen V, Pham TS, Vo CD, Le Thi QM, Ngo TT, Dao BK, Le Phuc P, Nguyen TT, Hoang TL, Cao VT, Le Truong G, Nguyen DT, Le Hong N, Nguyen Thi KT, Le Hoang S, Le Van T, Dolecek C, Tran TT, Jong MD, Schultsz C, Cheng P: Avian influenza A (H5N1) in 10 patients in Vietnam. New Engl J Med 2004;350:1179-1188.

25 Chotpitayasunondh T, Lochindarat S, Srisan P, Chokepaibulkit K, Weerakul J, Maneerattanaporn M, Sawanpanyalert P: Cases of influenza A (H5N1)—Thailand, 2004 (Reprinted from MMWR 2004;53:100-103). JAMA 2004;291:1059-1060.

26 Swayne DE, Beck JR: Experimental study to determine if low pathogenicity and high pathogenicity avian influenza viruses can be present in chicken breast and thigh meat following intranasal virus inoculation. Avian Dis 2005;49:81-85.

27 Tumpey TM, Suarez DL, Perkins LEL, Senne DA, Lee JG, Lee YJ, Mo IP, Sung HW, Swayne DE: Characterization of a highly pathogenic H5N1 avian influenza a virus isolated from duck meat. J Virol 2002;76:6344-6355.

28 Mase M, Eto M, Tanimura N, Imai K, Tsukamoto K, Horimoto T, Kawaoka Y, Yamaguchi S: Isolation of a genotypically unique H5N1 influenza virus from duck meat imported into Japan from China. Virology 2005;339:101-109.

29 Beato MS, Toffan A, De Nardi R, Cristalli A, Terregino C, Cattoli G, Capua I: A conventional, inactivated oil emulsion vaccine suppresses shedding and prevents viral meat colonisation in commercial (Pekin) ducks challenged with HPAI H5N1. Vaccine 2007;25:4064-4072.

Dr. David E. Swayne, Southeast Poultry Research Laboratory, USDA/Agricultural Research Service, 934 College Station Road, Athens, Georgia 30605, USA
E-mail: David.Swayne@ars.usda.gov

Dodet B and the Scientific & Technical Department of the OIE (eds): Vaccination: A Tool for the Control of Avian Influenza. Dev Biol (Basel). Basel, Karger, 2007, vol 130, p 133.

Efficacy of Immunization in Different Poultry Species

G. Koch

Central Institute of Animal Disease Control, Lelystad WUR, Netherlands

Keywords: avian influenza, vaccination, vaccine, biosecurity, poultry

Avian influenza is a devastating disease of poultry and is also a threat to public health, as new influenza viruses might emerge that cause a new influenza pandemic in humans. Biosecurity measures form the first line of defence against the introduction and subsequent spread of influenza viruses; however, biosecurity is hampered by the complexity of the poultry industry and the ways in which poultry are kept in some regions.

Vaccination is considered to be an additional method to complement biosecurity measures. Although vaccination cannot prevent virus introduction, it can and should reduce the spread of virus to levels at which, on average, one infected individual infects less than one other individual or, at the population level, one infected flock infects less than one other flock. Routinely, vaccination efficacy is tested on the basis of disease, mortality and virus shedding in vaccination challenge experiments. These experiments do not, however, take into account important epidemiological parameters such as infectious period, transmissibility, virulence and host resistance. To obtain estimates of these parameters, we have studied the transmission characteristics of highly pathogenic avian influenza viruses. In a transmission experiment, a certain number of infected birds are kept with a number of uninfected contact birds, and the infection chain is monitored by virus isolation and serology. Our results show that vaccination can reduce the transmission level to such an extent that a major outbreak can be prevented, depending on the time between challenge and vaccination and bird species, among other variables.

Dr. Guus Koch, Central Institute for Animal Disease Control Lelystad CIDC-Lelystad, Department of Virology, Po Box 2004, 8203 AA Lelystad, The Netherlands
E-mail: guus.koch@wur.nl

Dodet B and the Scientific & Technical Department of the OIE (eds): Vaccination: A Tool for the Control of Avian Influenza. Dev Biol (Basel). Basel, Karger, 2007, vol 130, pp 135-141.

Diagnosing Avian Influenza Infection in Vaccinated Populations by Systems for Differentiating Infected from Vaccinated Animals (DIVA)

I. Capua, G. Cattoli

OIE, FAO and National Reference Laboratory for Newcastle Disease and Avian Influenza, Istituto Zooprofilattico Sperimentale delle Venezie, Legnaro, Padova, Italy

Keywords: Diagnosis, avian influenza, vaccination, DIVA

Summary: Vaccination against avian influenza is recommended as a tool to support control measures in countries affected by avian influenza. Vaccination is known to increase the resistance of susceptible birds to infection and also to reduce shedding; however, it does not always prevent infection. Vaccinated infected flocks can therefore be a source of infection and thus be responsible for the perpetuation of infection.

To avoid the spread of infection in a vaccinated population, immunization strategies must allow differentiation of infected from vaccinated animals (DIVA), combined with an appropriate monitoring system. Vaccinated exposed flocks must be identified and managed by restriction policies that include controlled marketing and stamping-out. Several vaccines and diagnostic tests to detect infection in vaccinated populations are available, the tests having various properties and characteristics. In order to achieve eradication, the most appropriate DIVA vaccination strategy must be identified and an appropriate monitoring programme be designed, taking into account risk factors, the epidemiological situation and the socioeconomic implications of the policy.

Introduction

Avian influenza is one of the greatest concerns for public health that has emerged from the animal reservoir in recent times. Over the past 5 years, there has been a sharp increase in the number of outbreaks of avian influenza in poultry over that in the previous 40 years. It has been calculated that the impact of avian influenza on the poultry industry has increased 100-fold, with 23 million birds affected in the

40-year period between 1959 and 1998 and over 200 million between 1999 and 2006 [1]. In view of the low profile of avian influenza up to 1999, a significant amount of information and methods to manage avian influenza epidemics adequately are lacking. In particular, immunization against avian influenza in its notifiable form was discouraged until recently. As a result, studies and investments in avian influenza vaccinology have not been a priority, and we are facing an emergency with limited resources and experience.

Definition of Avian Influenza

The chapter on avian influenza in the *Terrestrial Code* of the OIE, which was enforced in January 2006 [2], represents the first modern approach to avian influenza, taking into account new scientific data on this disease and using it to regulate trade. The OIE adopted the following definition during its 73rd General Session:

"For the purposes of this *Terrestrial Code*, avian influenza in its notifiable form is defined as an infection of poultry caused by any influenza A virus of the H5 or H7 subtypes or by any avian influenza virus with an intravenous pathogenicity index greater than 1.2 (or as an alternative at least 75% mortality) as described below. Notifiable avian influenza viruses can be divided into highly pathogenic… and low-pathogenicity notifiable avian influenza viruses."

Another major change in the OIE code is that it introduces the concept of allowing the use of vaccination in avian populations from which commodities are derived that are destined for international trade. When these two concepts are combined, although infection with any virus of the H5 and H7 subtype or any other virus fulfilling the virulence criteria must be notified, the presence of antibodies as a result of vaccination does not limit international trade of commodities originating from these birds. With this in mind, immunization for notifiable avian influenza viruses must be approached from a wider angle.

Prevention of Avian Influenza

Primary introduction of avian influenza viruses into domestic poultry occurs through either direct or indirect contact with infected birds, which can happen during movement of infected poultry, movement of contaminated equipment, fomites or vehicles and penetration of contaminated infectious organic material. Airborne transmission over significant distances between farms has not been demonstrated to date. Therefore, avian influenza infections can be prevented if biosecurity measures are implemented at farm level. Outbreaks that involve significant numbers of animals are characterized by penetration of infection into the commercial circuit, including industrially reared poultry and also all other poultry that are traded, such as those from semi-intensive and backyard farms.

Biosecurity, encompassing bio-exclusion and bio-containment, is the first and most important means of prevention. It follows that if biosecurity measures of a high standard are implemented and maintained, they represent a firewall against penetration and perpetuation in the industrial circuit. Breaches in biosecurity systems do, however, occur. In such cases, the occurrence and extent of the breach should be evaluated and corrective measures follow, and they should be taken as an indication of the need for early warning systems and additional means of control against avian influenza, such as vaccines.

Currently Available Vaccines

Vaccines and companion diagnostic tests that allow application of the DIVA principle

Research in avian influenza vaccinology has only recently become a field of interest for pharmaceutical companies and research institutions. Therefore, the range of products and the performance of companion diagnostic tests is not adequate to fully cover the complex field situations associated with this infection.

Antigenic cross-reactivity between strains of the same haemagglutinin (H) subtype is believed to occur even between strains belonging to different lineages; however, it is not known how cross-protection is influenced by the immunological pressure generated by the variety of seed strains. Similarly, the occurrence and extent of antigenic drift in this situation is impossible to predict but could become a significant issue in the future.

At the time of writing, two types of vaccines were available on the market: inactivated vaccines based on adjuvanted whole virions and live recombinant vaccines. The former can be prepared from master seed viruses isolated during natural outbreaks, generated by reverse genetics or natural reassortants. Recombinant vector-based vaccines are engineered products based on a vector virus that expresses the haemagglutinin protein of avian influenza. Only fowl pox-vectored and a Newcastle disease-vectored vaccine are commercially available.

Whole virion vaccines and companion diagnostic tests or systems to reveal field exposure

These vaccines are based on a preparation containing inactivated virus grown in embryonated eggs or in cell culture. The seed strains that are currently being used include field isolates collected during natural outbreaks and viruses generated by reverse genetics technology. The former were prepared to face emergency situations, and the seed strains were selected without harmonized criteria. They may therefore contain seed viruses of high or low pathogenicity, although the OIE guidelines indicate that low-pathogenicity notifiable avian influenza strains should be used [2].

In inactivated reverse genetics-based vaccines [3,4], the seed strain is a synthetic virus, completely engineered in the laboratory. These viruses contain a backbone derived from a virus that has a high replication capacity (A/Puerto Rico/8/34 H1N1), with the two genes encoding for surface antigens (H and N) derived from contemporary viruses. The multi-basic cleavage site of the haemagglutinin gene (*HA*) of the high-pathogenicity donor virus is modified into a low-pathogenicity motif. This combination of genes allows excellent replicative efficiency, which ensures high-titre, consistent virus yields during production, and suitable surface antigens. As these vaccines have the same properties as conventional inactivated vaccines, the same companion tests can be used.

In order to be efficacious, inactivated conventional vaccines must contain a seed virus of the same haemagglutinin subtype as the field strain against which vaccination is directed, while the subtype of the other surface antigen, the neuraminidase (N) protein, is virtually irrelevant with regard to protection [5]. Thus, vaccines can contain a seed virus of the same subtype as the field strain (H5N1 vaccine to combat an

H5N1 field challenge) or can be of the same H subtype but with a different N (H5N9 vaccine to combat an H5N1 field challenge). The latter is known as heterologous vaccination.

Two methods for detecting exposure with this type of vaccine have been evaluated in the field, with satisfactory results. Unvaccinated sentinels have been used to identify field exposure within a vaccinated population, regardless of the strain used in the vaccine. This system requires identification of unvaccinated birds and regular clinical inspection, in conjunction with serological testing to detect low-pathogenicity notifiable avian influenza; highly pathogenic notifiable avian influenza is clearly seen as clinical disease in the sentinel birds. The system is deemed to be valid but is impractical, particularly when birds not confined to cages have to be identified within a flock. Furthermore, there is a risk that sentinel birds could be replaced by naive birds in order to escape restriction policies.

In heterologous vaccination, the diversity between the N antigen in the vaccine and that in the field can be used as a natural marker system. This system, known as the 'differentiation of infected from vaccinated animals' (DIVA) system, was developed in Italy in 2001 and has been used to combat many introductions of notifiable avian influenza [6]. The system is based on the detection of antibodies to the N protein of the field virus, which provide evidence of field infection. Currently, only an indirect immunofluorescent antibody test has been fully validated [7,8], although a competitive ELISA test is undergoing preliminary validation [9,10].

A promising system that could be used as a companion test to vaccines containing homologous or heterologous seed strains is based on detection of anti-NS1 antibodies [11]. The system is based on the fact that the NS1 protein is synthesized only during active viral replication and is therefore not present in significant amounts when inactivated vaccines, which do not replicate in birds, are used. Birds vaccinated with such vaccines develop antibodies to the NS1 only after field exposure. Full and field validation of this system under various circumstances is still in progress [12] and should be completed before this system is recommended. No diagnostic kit has been validated to date.

Recombinant vaccines and companion tests

Recombinant vaccines are based on expression of the HA protein of avian influenza in a vector virus or another system and include recombinant live vectored vaccines and recombinant protein-based vaccines.

Recombinant live vectored vaccines are based on insertion of an H5 or H7 haemagglutinin gene in a suitable replicating vector, which will, during replication, induce the production of antibodies to the haemagglutinin of the influenza gene. Fowl pox-based recombinant viruses have obtained marketing authorization and are being used in several countries. Newcastle disease virus-based recombinants have been designed by several groups [13,14], and a product developed by Chinese researchers is being used in the field in China. A product based on infectious laryngotracheitis virus has also been described [15]. These preparations, with the exception of that designed by Swayne et al. [13], offer protection against clinical signs and reduce shedding. They can elicit immunity in the presence of maternally derived antibodies [16] but the efficacy of most of these products in the presence of pre-existing antibodies due to natural infection with a field strain of the vector virus, such as Newcastle disease virus or fowl poxvirus, remains to be established [17].

The greatest advantage of these products is that companion diagnostic tests for antibodies to any viral proteins other than the haemagglutinin can be used to identify field-exposed flocks. Thus, agar gel immunodiffusion or ELISA tests for antibodies to NP or M proteins can be used, allowing detection of a field challenge with any influenza A virus. Tests for the detection of antibodies to the N protein can be used to identify field exposure only to viruses of known N subtype.

Recombinant protein-based vaccines are synthesized in the laboratory by expression of the haemagglutinin in a suitable system, for example baculoviruses, plants or yeasts [18]. Several prototypes have been developed and tested in the laboratory, with encouraging results; however, probably because of the cost of production, they have not attracted commercial interest. Use of any of these 'engineered' vaccines in the field would have several advantages, including the availability of a variety of companion diagnostic tests, as for recombinant vectored vaccines, and updating the haemagglutinin component, should this be required.

In summary, to date, only conventional inactivated (containing natural or synthetic strains) and recombinant live vectored vaccines are available for use, coupled with suitable companion diagnostic tests. Both have advantages and limitations for application in the field, and more research is needed to optimize the products and their companion tests in order to tackle the problem of avian influenza, in view of its complexity and spread.

Conclusions

The epidemiology of avian influenza infection has changed during the past decade because of the persistence and continuous spread of H5N1 HPAI among domestic poultry populations in vast geographical areas of three continents and because of the marked increase in the number of outbreaks of avian influenza worldwide. Furthermore, H5N1 can spread to previously unaffected areas; its recent isolation from apparently healthy migratory birds in southern China suggests that they can contribute to virus transmission over long distances during migration [19]. This unprecedented situation could represent a threat of H5N1 virus introduction or re-emergence in domestic poultry populations worldwide, with inauspicious and unpredictable consequences.

Vaccination including the DIVA system, in conjunction with a territorial strategy, could be successful in controlling and eradicating avian influenza infections in poultry and could make possible the continuation of international trade. Its management is, however, complex and might include failures, such as the spread of infection in a vaccinated population. Vaccination programmes must therefore be based on a suitable product, which allows the detection of field-exposed flocks, and with a monitoring system to guarantee early detection of and rapid response to avian influenza. For this reason, international organizations responsible for trade regulations and animal disease control should establish a set of guidelines to 'accredit' control programmes for international recognition. Such a policy would have several practical advantages, resulting in improved crisis management, including harmonization of the seed viruses to be used in vaccines, rapid approval of established control programmes, constant updating of the field situation, feedback of information on successes and failures, harmonization of protocols and systems and public availability of control and eradication programmes. In this way, even developing countries in which there are notifiable avian influenza infections and that have no experience with avian influenza management can use previous experience to combat this infection in an educated manner, thus avoiding wastage of resources and time. Harmonizing programmes and sharing information would also lead to better knowledge about the epidemiology of notifiable avian influenza infections, which would enhance management skills, including the identification of reservoir species.

Vaccination is now being used extensively in preventing the introduction of or controlling widespread H5N1 HPAI. The veterinary community has limited first-hand experience in managing this disease with the help of vaccination. Appropriate management will probably have positive results; however, errors will be made, and it is imperative that control and eradication processes benefit from the lessons derived from such errors. In addition, control programmes should be managed in a flexible and transparent manner to respond to the continuous challenges that avian influenza infections pose.

References

1 Capua I, Alexander DJ: Avian influenza: recent developments. Avian Pathol 2004;33:393-404.

2 OIE : Terrestrial Animal Code, chapter 14, 2.7.12.1. Paris, World Organisation for Animal Health, 2005 www.oie.int/eng/normes/mcode/en_chapter_2.7.12.htm.

3 Tian G, Zhang S, Li Y, Bu Z, Liu P, Zhou J, Li C, Shi J, Yu K, Chen H: Protective efficacy in chickens, geese and ducks of an H5N1-inactivated vaccine developed by reverse genetics. Virology 2005;341(1):153-162.

4 Webster RG, Webby RJ, Hoffmann E, Rodenberg J, Kumar M, Seiler P, Krauss S, Songserm T: The immunogenicity and efficacy against H5N1 challenge of reverse genetics-derived H5N3 influenza vaccine in ducks and chickens. Virology 2006;351:303-311.

5 Swayne DE, Perdue ML, Beck JR, Garcia M, Suarez DL: Vaccines protect chickens against H5 highly pathogenic avian influenza in the face of genetic changes in field viruses over multiple years. Vet Microbiol 2000;74:165-172.

6 Capua I, Marangon S: The use of vaccination to combat multiple introductions of notifiable avian influenza viruses of the H5 an H7 subtypes between 2000 and 2006 in Italy. Vaccine 2007; 25:4987-4995.

7 Cattoli G, Terregino C, Brasola V, Rodriguez JF, Capua I: Development and preliminary validation of an ad hoc N1–N3 discriminatory test for the control of avian influenza in Italy. Avian Dis 2003; 47(Suppl 3):1060-1062.

8 Cattoli G, Milani A, Bettini F, Beato MS, Mancin M, Terregino C, Capua I: Development and validation of an anti-N3 indirect immunofluorescent antibody test to be used as a companion diagnostic test in the framework of a 'DIVA' vaccination strategy for avian influenza infections in poultry. Avian Pathol 2006;35:154-159.

9 Dundon WG, Terregino C, Tuttoilmondo V, Pizzuto M, Busani L, Mancin M, Cattoli G, Capua I: Preliminary validation of a commercial avian influenza N1 antibody competitive ELISA test that can be used as a part of DIVA strategy. In: Epizone First Annual Meeting, 30 May-1 June 2007, Pulawy, Poland. Lelystad, Centraal Instituut voor Dierziekte Controle, 2007.

10 Pourquier P, Lesceu S: Avian influenza DIVA testing: preliminary validation of a commercial competitive ELISA for N1 antibodies in bird sera. In: Book of abstracts. FAO/OIE Conference on Vaccination: A Tool for the Control of Avian Influenza, Verona, 2007. Rome, Food and Agricultural Organization of the United Nations, 2007, pp 75-76.

11 Tumpey TM, Alvarez R, Swayne DE, Suarez DL: Diagnostic approach for differentiating infected from vaccinated poultry on the basis of antibodies to NS1, the nonstructural protein of influenza A virus. J Clin Microbiol 2005;43:676-683.

12 Dundon W, Maniero S, Toffan A, Capua I, Cattoli G: Appearance of serum antibodies against the avian influenza non-structural 1 protein in experimentally infected chickens and turkeys. Avian Dis 2007;51(Suppl 1):209-12.

13 Swayne DE, Suarez DL, Schultz-Cherry S, Tumpey TM, King DJ, Nakaya T, Palese P, Garcia-Sastre A: Recombinant paramyxovirus type 1-avian influenza-H7 virus as a vaccine for protection of chickens against influenza and Newcastle disease. Avian Dis 2003;47(Suppl 3):1047-1050.

14 Veits J, Wiesner D, Fuchs W, Hoffmann B, Granzow H, Starick E, Mundt E, Schirrmeier H, Mebatsion T, Mettenleiter TC, Romer-Oberdorfer A: Newcastle disease virus expressing H5 hemagglutinin gene protects chickens against Newcastle disease and avian influenza. Proc Natl Acad Sci USA 2006;103:8197-8202.

15 Luschow D, Werner O, Mettenleiter TC, Fuchs W: Protection of chickens from lethal avian influenza A virus infection by live-virus vaccination with infectious laryngotracheitis virus recombinants expressing the hemagglutinin (H5) gene. Vaccine 2001;19:4249-4259.

16 Bublot M, Pritchard N, Swayne DE, Selleck P, Karaca K, Suarez DL, Audonnet JC, Mickle TR: Development and use of fowlpox vectored vaccines for avian influenza. Ann N York Acad Sci 2006; 1081:193-201.

17 Swayne DE, Beck JR, Kinney N: Failure of a recombinant fowl poxvirus vaccine containing an avian influenza hemagglutinin gene to provide consistent protection against influenza in chickens preimmunized with a fowl pox vaccine. Avian Dis 2000;44:132-137.

18 Swayne DE: Application of new vaccine technologies for the control of transboundary diseases. Dev Biol (Basel) 2004;119:219-228.

19 Chen H, Smith GJ, Zhang SY, Qin K, Wang J, Li KS, Webster RG, Peiris JS, Guan Y: Avian flu: H5N1 virus outbreak in migratory waterfowl. Nature 2005;436:191-192.

Dr. Ilaria Capua, OIE, FAO and National Reference Laboratory for Newcastle Disease and Avian Influenza, Istituto Zooprofilattico Sperimentale delle Venezie, Viale dell'Università 10, 35020 Legnaro, Padova, Italy
E-mail: icapua@izsvenezie.it

Dodet B and the Scientific & Technical Department of the OIE (eds): Vaccination: A Tool for the Control of Avian Influenza. Dev Biol (Basel). Basel, Karger, 2007, vol 130, p 143.

SESSION VI

Regulatory and Trade Aspects

Chairperson: *D.E. Swayne,* USA

Dodet B and the Scientific & Technical Department of the OIE (eds): Vaccination: A Tool for the Control of Avian Influenza. Dev Biol (Basel). Basel, Karger, 2007, vol 130, p 145.

Legal Aspects of Vaccination of Poultry against Avian Influenza in the European Union

M. Pittman

European Commission, Directorate General Health and Consumer Protection, Brussels, Belgium

Keywords: EU directive, avian influenza, poultry vaccination

In the European Union, the new Council Directive 2005/94/EC on the control of avian influenza allows implementation not only of emergency (short-term) vaccination after a disease outbreak but also of preventive (long-term) vaccination plans. The European Union Member States must base their decision to vaccinate on the outcome of a risk assessment in which risk factors for the introduction and spread of infection to poultry and other captive birds are identified, such as the occurrence of an outbreak on its territory or in a neighbouring country, the location of the poultry in areas close to wetlands, where migratory birds gather and the types of husbandry systems.

Member States must submit a vaccination plan for approval by the Commission and must impose certain restrictions on the movement of vaccinated birds. In order to detect virus circulation in vaccinated birds, vaccination must be coupled with monitoring and active surveillance schemes, which should follow the differentiation of infected from vaccinated animals (DIVA) strategy.

Dr. Maria Pittman, European Commission, rue Froissart 101, Office 3/84, Brussels 1049, Belgium
E-mail : maria.pittman@ec.europa.eu

Dodet B and the Scientific & Technical Department of the OIE (eds): Vaccination: A Tool for the Control of Avian Influenza. Dev Biol (Basel). Basel, Karger, 2007, vol 130, p 147.

SESSION VII

Vaccination: an Integrated Approach

Chairperson: *A. Laddomada,* European Commission

Dodet B and the Scientific & Technical Department of the OIE (eds): Vaccination: A Tool for the Control of Avian Influenza. Dev Biol (Basel). Basel, Karger, 2007, vol 130, pp 149-156.

The Vaccination Programme in Indonesia

E. Sawitri Siregar[1], Darminto[2], J. Weaver[3], A. Bouma[4]

1 Coordinator, Avian Influenza Campaign Management Unit, Ministry of Agriculture, Ragunan Jakarta Selatan, Indonesia

2 Director, Research Institute for Veterinary Science, Ministry of Agriculture, Ragunan Jakarta Selatan, Indonesia

3 Senior Technical Advisor, FAO, Jakarta, Indonesia

4 Faculty of Veterinary Medicine, Utrecht University, Netherlands

Keywords: HPAI, poultry, vaccination, Indonesia

Summary: The Indonesian response to the outbreak of highly pathogenic avian influenza (HPAI) is being strengthened by increased intersectoral commitment and greater availability of staff and resources. Vaccination against avian influenza has been used widely in large commercial sectors but less so in other sectors. Generally, there has been a reduction in outbreaks and in the impact of HPAI on the commercial industry. A field trial is described that might provide insight into the efficacy of vaccination on farms in sector 3. Preliminary data suggest that vaccination of layers induces high titres, whereas vaccination of native chickens might be difficult owing to a low response in these breeds. A much greater commitment of management, staff and resources is required before vaccination can become part of a successful sustainable campaign to eradicate HPAI. For success, the commercial poultry industry must become an integral part of the control programme, providing information and having the opportunity to identify or modify the priorities of the control programme.

Background

Indonesia is a large, complex archipelago with diverse ethnic groups, religious beliefs and cultures. The human population is now estimated to be over 240 million, of whom more than 60% live on Java. More than 6000 islands are inhabited. Indonesia has adopted a decentralized system of government, currently with 33 provinces and 444 districts, which have high levels of local autonomy.

Indonesia has an estimated annual poultry population of 1.5 billion. The poultry industry is diverse, ranging from the industrial sector to free-ranging village production, and includes chickens, ducks, muscovy ducks, quail and geese. The standing population is some 600 million, with 300 million chickens in sector 4 villages (*ayam kampung*), 165 million broilers, 100 million layers and 35 million ducks. The poultry population mirrors the human population, with more than 65% in Java, particularly concentrated in western Java around Jakarta.

The first outbreaks of highly pathogenic avian influenza (HPAI) occurred in mid-2003, with formal confirmation of H5N1 in January 2004. An epidemic of HPAI has since spread across much of the country, overwhelming efforts at control. HPAI is now endemic in much of Java, Sumatra, Bali and South Sulawesi, with outbreaks also occurring elsewhere. HPAI outbreaks have now been confirmed in 30 of the 33 provinces. Since July 2005, human cases have been confirmed repeatedly in Indonesia, and the largest number of human fatalities in the world due to H5N1 have occurred in this country.

Government Programme

The Government of Indonesia introduced a policy of vaccination as part of its nine-point plan for the eradication of HPAI in June 2004. The policy states that all poultry are to be vaccinated within 6 months, followed by routine vaccination. Since its introduction, the vaccination policy has been that poultry in sectors 3 and 4 are vaccinated under a Government programme at no cost to the owners; the commercial sector undertakes its own vaccination programmes at its cost. Sector 3 is covered only up to a maximum of 5000 birds.

Indonesia has a formal process of drug and vaccine registration. Since introduction of the policy of vaccination against avian influenza, 11 vaccines have been registered, including H5N1, H5N2 and H5N9 seed strains, and several others are undergoing registration, including a recombinant pox vaccine.

Initially, the Government programme used locally produced H5N1 vaccines from an Indonesian virus seed strain. In early 2006, the policy was changed to use of a low-pathogenicity avian influenza virus seed strain. The two Indonesian manufacturers of avian influenza vaccine currently have H5N2 vaccines under registration, and the Government purchased imported H5N2 vaccines for its programme in 2006. The Government has thus purchased vaccine since 2004, in an attempt to meet its policy objective, but supplies and delivery logistics have been inadequate. The scale of the task is immense: if it is assumed that all 300 million birds in sector 4 are to be vaccinated twice to achieve effective immunity and that these birds have an average lifespan of 6 months, then 1.2 billion doses must be given annually, if one were to target the whole population. The amount of Government-supplied vaccine was 132 million doses in 2004, 143 million in 2005 and 55 million in 2006.

In addition to the problem of availability of vaccine, there are huge logistic problems in delivering this extensive vaccination programme. These problems and the task of administering vaccine to free-ranging birds, have resulted in limited vaccine coverage. Under the Government programme, vaccine has been administered by the district livestock services (*Dinas Peternakan*). Poor biosecurity during administration of vaccine and lack of understanding about incubation periods have sometimes resulted in further spread of disease and also created a loss of public confidence in the benefits of vaccination.

Vaccine use is audited by the Ministry of Agriculture, which assesses usage rates against populations: these rarely exceed 30% and may be much lower. Researchers have investigated the immune response with haemagglutination inhibition tests at a number of locations and over time. Considerable research has been carried out on the immune levels achieved with different vaccination regimens. Table 1 shows the benefit of repeated vaccination in raising the geometric mean titre. Table 2 shows the percentage of birds with titres $\geq {}^2\log 4$ measured at various Government disease investigation centres.

Table 1: Antibody titres in vaccinated breeders, Indonesia

Time	**No. of samples**	**GMT (HI-$\log^2$)**
After first vaccination	34	3.1
After second vaccination	15	7.2
After third vaccination	40	7.5

From RIVS, Bogor

Table 2: Birds with titre $\geq {}^2\log 4$, by type and Disease Investigation Centre (DIC) in Indonesia

District	**Purebred chickens**		**Native chickens**	
	Protected[a] (%) (n)	Unprotected (%) (n)	Protected[a] (%) (n)	Unprotected (%) (n)
Medan	78 (647)	22 (22)	61 (685)	40 (443)
Wates	55 (609)	45 (500)	20 (179)	80 (730)
Bali	33 (176)	67 (352)	11 (46)	89 (364)
Maros	80 (1658)	20 (406)	–	–

[a] $\geq {}^2\log 4$

Ring vaccination is used as part of the response to an HPAI outbreak whenever possible. The vaccine used is supplied by the Government and is currently imported H5N2 vaccine. Constraints to the use of vaccine in an outbreak are that it is not always possible to define a 'safe' population in an endemically infected area to conduct ring vaccination, and vaccine supplies are not always available. There is also obvious concern about inadequate levels of biosecurity and the possibility of further spread of HPAI or other diseases.

Commercial Industry Programmes

The initial HPAI epidemic affected commercial industry, with significant numbers of bird deaths, destocking costs and decreased demand, with reduced prices. Government figures indicate that by the end of 2006, some 11 million poultry had died from HPAI, and a further 8 million were culled.

The commercial industry has adopted a range of vaccination programmes with a number of different vaccines. The programmes appear to have reduced losses, but outbreaks are known to continue in the commercial sector. The protocols vary by company but in general include:

- vaccination of grandparent and parent layer flocks four times up to the point of lay, with one or two boosters;

- vaccination of layers two to three times to the point of lay and sometimes one booster;
- no vaccination of broilers, except in identified high-risk areas where they receive a half dose at day 7; and
- checking of immune levels every 4-5 weeks by the haemagglutination inhibition test.

Companies manage the health of their poultry with vaccination against the usual range of diseases, including Newcastle disease, infectious bursal disease, infectious bronchitis, coryza, infectious laryngotracheitis, reovirus, egg drop syndrome, fowl pox and cocci. Unusual flock deaths are investigated, samples commonly being submitted to company laboratories. The laboratory facilities vary but can have the capability to conduct conventional polymerase chain reaction (PCR) and virus isolation.

Commercial companies are concerned about the variable immunogenicity of the registered vaccines and their inability to protect broilers effectively with the current killed vaccines. They would like to have improved, innovative vaccines, such as the recombinant pox vaccine for use in day-old chicks and Newcastle disease-vectored H5 vaccines. Some companies conduct their own 'challenge testing' to assess vaccine performance.

Field Vaccination Pilot Study

Within the Dutch–Indonesia Sukabumi Project, a field trial was conducted to determine the efficacy of locally produced vaccines [3]. Only sector 3 flocks were included in the trial, which consisted of one treatment group and one control group. The treatment group comprised one layer farm and four semi-intensive native chicken flocks; the control group comprised three layer and two semi-intensive native chicken farms. The treated flocks were vaccinated twice with a local homologous vaccine, either by their own farm staff or by officers of the livestock services. All native chickens in a 1-km ring around each treatment flock were also vaccinated. In the control flocks, the usual vaccination programme and vaccines were used, but no ring vaccination was carried out. The vaccine coverage and the titres of haemagglutinin antibodies are being monitored regularly in serum samples taken before vaccination, at the second vaccination and either at 4 weeks after vaccination (layer flocks) or at the end of production (3 weeks after the second vaccination) in semi-intensive native chicken flocks.

Surveillance for virus circulation in this field trial was based on the 'differentiating infected from vaccinated animals' (DIVA) principle, by using sentinels in all 10 flocks in the trial. The sentinels were from a commercial layer farm; they were not vaccinated against avian influenza but were vaccinated against other viral diseases according to the regular schedule. The sentinels were monitored serologically to detect circulation of low-pathogenicity strains of avian influenza. If sentinels died or became sick, tracheal and cloacal swab samples were taken, which were subsequently tested by PCR to detect the presence of HPAI H5 strains. Use of sentinels makes it possible to interpret positive serological results as vaccination-induced titres, as long as the sentinels remain healthy and seronegative.

Farmers appeared to be reluctant to accept the introduction of sentinels into their flocks. Preliminary monitoring of vaccination-induced antibody titres showed that

75% of the layers in the treatment group on the layer farm seroconverted after the second vaccination and had titres of ^{2}log 5 or higher (see Table 3). In a second sample from another shed on the same farm, all birds had seroconverted after two vaccinations. This finding indicates that a double vaccination with a local vaccine should be sufficient to induce antibody titres and a coverage that can be assumed to reduce virus shedding. In the four native chicken farms in the treatment group, the coverage of birds with a titre $\geq^{2}$log 4 was on average 15-40% after two vaccinations, and the average titre in seroconverted birds was lower. These findings indicate that the immune response is probably not sufficient to prevent further spread of the virus. The results for samples collected on control layer farms included in the trial are not yet available. The titres in the various flocks are shown in Table 3. As the sentinels were seronegative, the titres were proably due to vaccination.

Table 3: Serological data from the vaccination field trial in Indonesia

Group	Percentage birds with ^{2}log $\geq$ 4	Range of titres ^{2}log
Treated		
Layers	75	5-11
Native chicken farms	15, 15, 25, 40[a]	4-5
Native chickens (ring)	58, 65, 60[b]	0-4
Control		
Layers	Not Determined	
Native chicken farms	20, 80[c]	4-7
Native chickens (ring)	0	0

[a] Data for four flocks
[b] Data from three areas (rings)
[c] Data for two flocks

The preliminary results show that the DIVA principle, with sentinels, was successfully implemented and is essential for interpreting serological data on immune status. Double vaccination of layers appeared to induce titres > ^{2}log 4 against H5, but it was difficult to achieve high titres in native chickens. Sentinels are necessary to determine whether (subclinical) outbreaks can occur in flocks vaccinated with homologous vaccines or in flocks given a heterologous vaccine when no differentiating diagnostic tests are available. Use of sentinels can show whether vaccines are effective in preventing outbreaks of H5N1. These surveillance data are not yet available. As only a limited number of flocks were included in this study, a sound statistical analysis is not possible, and the results cannot be extrapolated.

A Phased Progressive Control Programme

The Government, supported by a number of international donors, has considerably strengthened its operational capacity to combat HPAI. A critical component of the next phase will be progressive introduction by region of blanket vaccination, with more rigorous application of other necessary control measures, such as increased public awareness and commitment, early detection and response, improved biosecurity at markets and for dealers, movement control and a reduction in the threat from waterfowl. Greater emphasis will be placed on stopping human exposure by ensuring rapid culling in the case of outbreaks on infected farms and reducing virus transmission by improving village, poultry enterprise and market biosecurity.

It is also critical to the success of the HPAI control programme that the problem be addressed in the commercial poultry industry, the concerns of which must be considered. The requirements include their formal commitment to HPAI control, recognition of the need to exchange information on the disease situation, improved biosecurity and the use of best-practice vaccination programmes, with monitoring and evaluation to assess efficacy and the presence of circulating viruses.

The proposed blanket vaccination campaign will be limited in time. A series of phased regional operations is envisaged to eliminate infection from island groups. Priority will be given to areas in which the highest numbers of human cases have occurred, primarily in western Java (Banten, West Java and Jakarta provinces).

The proposed Phase 1 will be a short preparatory period of 4–6 months, leading into a full control programme of targeted vaccination, initially in Bali. This will be extended into West Java and Banten at the earliest opportunity, most probably after a further 6 months. This phase will benefit from the experience gained and allow funding and resource commitments to be established. There will be no policy of blanket vaccination in Jakarta owing to the recent ban on poultry keeping. In further phases, the proposed programme will extend from the initial targeted areas: phase 2 in eastern Java, phase 3 in central Java and then further progressive phases, as resources permit. Fig. 1 shows the proposed phased campaign for implementing aggressive control measures with blanket vaccination to eliminate HPAI.

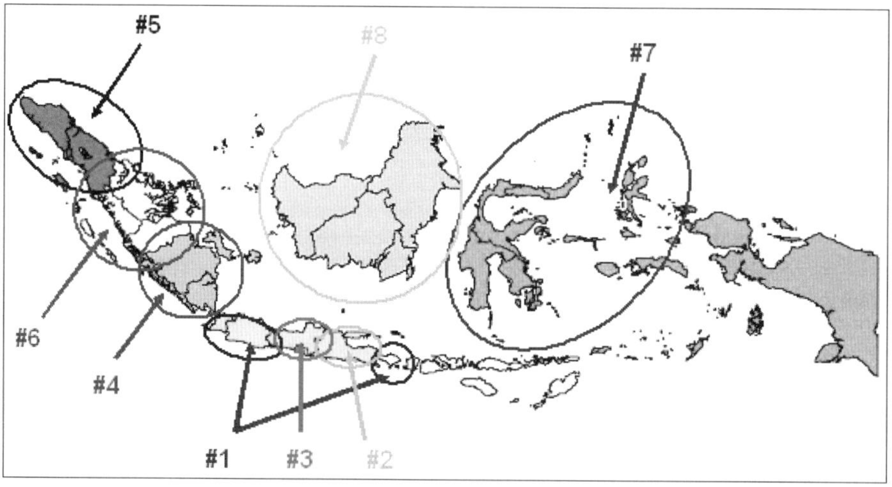

Fig. 1: Phased programme for aggressive control measures with blanket vaccination in Indonesia

The first phase will be undertaken as proof of principle. From the outset, care will be taken to create a system for measuring key indicators of success in programme delivery and disease control; progress in control will be assessed by the ability to deliver vaccine effectively and by assessment of disease incidence. A robust schedule of evaluation and monitoring will be built into the programme. Lack of investment or of demonstrable progress will lead to the whole programme being abandoned or modified.

The cost of a programme, such as this, are high. A model designed by FAO [1] indicates that the annual costs of vaccinating flocks in sectors 3 and 4 would be US$ 4.5 million in Bali and US$ 25 million in Banten and West Java.

Targeted vaccination will be conducted by various mechanisms, involving local governments, participatory disease response teams, lay and community vaccinators, private veterinarians and non-governmental organizations. All vaccinators will be trained. It is proposed that all poultry except broilers will be vaccinated in two rounds of two vaccinations per year. Broilers will be vaccinated with a recombinant pox vaccine as day-old chicks or with an inactivated vaccine at 7 days. In particular, all ducks will be vaccinated. Vaccination will be offered to the owners of fighting cocks, and they will be encouraged to participate in vaccination programmes. Pigeons, doves and ornamental birds will not be vaccinated.

The poultry industry will be required to conduct appropriate vaccination procedures on their premises, and checks will be conducted. All hatcheries supplying campaign areas will be required to vaccinate day-old chicks and ducklings according to agreed protocols.

The scale of the task of blanket vaccination of village chickens and smaller producers (sectors 3 and 4) should not be underestimated. The Brandenburg model was used to calculate the costs of the national campaign, for an average district and for Java district [2] (Table 4).

Table 4: Estimates of costs of vaccination programme from a model

Cost	**Average district, national**	**Average district, Java**	**Indonesia**
Number of sector 4 chickens	675 000	1 688 000	297 000 000
Number of sector 3 chickens	300 000	750 000	132 000 000
Number of ducks	38 000	94 000	16 500 000
Total poultry population	1 013 000	2 532 000	445 500 000
Vaccination equipment	39 000	98 000	17 271 000
Vaccine cost	46 000	114 000	20 041 000
Vaccinators' salaries	138 000	346 000	60 894 000
Post-vaccination monitoring	55 000	137 000	24 176 000
Government infrastructure	26 000	66 000	11 598 000
Cold storage	24 000	60 000	10 612 000
Communications	50 000	125 000	22 000 000
Number of vaccinators needed	350	875	154 000
Total number of poultry to vaccinate	1 013 000	2 531 000	445 500 000
Total vaccination cost per year	379 000	947 000	166 593 000

Population statistics taken from the Ministry of Agriculture's annual report [2].

Conclusion

The Indonesian response to the HPAI outbreak is being strengthened by greater use of vaccination against avian influenza. The field trial is providing insight into the efficacy of vaccination on sector 3 farms. For HPAI control to be successful, greater commitment of management, staff and resources is required before vaccination can become part of a successful, sustainable campaign for eradication of avian influenza. The commercial poultry industry must also become an integral part of the control programme.

References

1 Brandenburg B: Vaccination costing model. Unpublished document. Rome, Food and Agricultural Organisation of the United Nations, 2007.

2 Statistik Peternakan: Direktorat Jenderal Peternakan Departemen Pertanian RI, Edisi, Jakarta 2006.

3 Sukabumi Livestock Services, Dinas Peternakan Sukabumi, CIVAS, Wageningen International Field vaccination trial progress report June-December 2006.

Dr. Elly Sawitri Siregar, Coordinator, Avian Influenza Campaign Management Unit, Ministry of Agriculture, Republic of Indonesia; Directorate General of Livestock Services, Directorate of Animal Health, Jl. Harsono RM N°3 Building C, 9th Floor, Room 977, Jakarta, Indonesia
E-mail : elly@deptan.go.id; upp_ai@yahoo.com

Dodet B and the Scientific & Technical Department of the OIE (eds): Vaccination: A Tool for the Control of Avian Influenza. Dev Biol (Basel). Basel, Karger, 2007, vol 130, pp 157-158.

Control of Avian Influenza: a Vaccination Approach in Viet Nam

T.L. To[1], Q.A. Bui[1], N.H. Dau[1], V.N. Hoang[1], D.K. Van[1], N. Taylor[2], H.D. Do[1]

1 Department of Animal Health, Ministry of Agriculture and Rural Development, Hanoi, Viet Nam

2 PAN Livestock Services Ltd, Veterinary Epidemiology and Economics Research Unit, University of Reading, Reading, United Kingdom

Keywords: HPAI, avian influenza, immunization, Viet Nam

The first cases of highly pathogenic avian influenza were confirmed in Viet Nam in December 2003 in the north of the country and then in almost all provinces, with 24% of communes and 60% of towns affected at the peak of the epidemic. By March 2004, 45 million birds (17% of the poultry population) had died or been culled. A national vaccination programme was undertaken from October 2005 for all chickens and ducks. Post-vaccination serological monitoring and virus surveillance were organized to assess the immune response and to detect virus circulation.

No outbreaks of avian influenza occurred between December 2005 and December 2006. The coverage of the first round of vaccination was 66% of thc census population of chickens and almost 80% of ducks, and 67% of birds sampled at 1 or 2 months post-vaccination had positive haemagglutinin titres. Coverage was lower in the second round, 60% having positive haemagglutinin titres. After the two rounds of vaccination, > 70% of sampled birds in 55% of tested flocks had positive haemagglutinin titres. The coverage in the third campaign was 50% of chickens and more than 70% of ducks. Coverage in closed breeding farms was 100%, and the compliance rate was > 75%. This indicates the difficulty of ensuring a high percentage of immune individuals in a large and changing poultry population. The results of virus surveillance indicated that highly pathogenic viruses continue to circulate in waterfowl, especially in the south, presenting a permanent risk for infection of domestic poultry, as confirmed by outbreaks in late 2006 and early 2007 in some southern provinces.

In conclusion, the fact that there were no outbreaks of avian influenza in 2006 strongly suggests that the epidemic was controlled by positive measures, including mass immunization.

Dr.Thanh Long To, PAN Livestock Services Ltd, Veterinary Epidemiology and Economics Research Unit, University of Reading, Reading, UK
National Center for Veterinary Diagnosis, Department of Animal Health, Ministry of Agriculture and Rural Development, 11, Lane 78, Giai Phong Street, Hanoi 84 4, Viet Nam
E-mail: thanto@fpt.vn and tznt2002@yahoo.com

Dodet B and the Scientific & Technical Department of the OIE (eds): Vaccination: A Tool for the Control of Avian Influenza. Dev Biol (Basel). Basel, Karger, 2007, vol 130, p 159.

SESSION VIII

Conclusions and Recommendations

Chairperson: *B. Vallat, OIE,* France

Dodet B and the Scientific & Technical Department of the OIE (eds): Vaccination: A Tool for the Control of Avian Influenza. Dev Biol (Basel). Basel, Karger, 2007, vol 130, pp 161-165.

Recommendations

The conference on 'Vaccination: a Tool for the Control of Avian Influenza', organized by the World Organisation for Animal Health, the Food and Agriculture Organization of the United Nations and the Istituto Zooprofilattico Sperimentale delle Venezie, supported and co-organized by the European Commission and held in Verona, Italy, 20-22 March 2007,

CONSIDERING:

- the occurrence and dynamics of H5N1 in the current epizootic of highly pathogenic avian influenza (HPAI);
- the standards, guidelines and recommendations of the World Organisation for Animal Health (OIE), the guidelines and recommendations of the Food and Agriculture Organization of the United Nations (FAO) and the FAO-OIE global strategy on HPAI;
- experience with programmes for the control of avian influenza in countries and regions such as Italy, Mexico and South-East Asia;
- the successful control of HPAI outbreaks with vaccination as one of the critical measures in countries such as Viet Nam, Hong Kong SAR and other parts of China;
- the necessity of stopping the spread of H5N1 at the animal source and decreasing the risks for human infections and for the potential emergence of a human pandemic strain if detection, reporting or implementation of other control measures is delayed;
- the importance of disease awareness and surveillance programmes for early detection and early warning of infection;
- the experimental and field evidence that vaccination with high-quality, authorized vaccines increases resistance against infection, decreases the rate of excretion of the virus into the environment and in so doing decreases the probability of infection of poultry, other animals and humans;
- scientific advances in the development of novel vaccines against avian influenza that allow use of the 'differentiation of infected from vaccinated animals' (DIVA) concept and the accompanying diagnostic tools;
- that vaccination is not the only means available for controlling avian influenza, cannot eliminate the virus when used alone and, when used, must

be combined with other methods, such as culling of (potentially) infected animals, increased biosecurity at farm, household and market levels and movement control;

- that vaccination is logistically demanding and costly, with inherent uncertainties under field conditions with regard to the level and duration of protection against infection;
- that the overall aim should be not to rely on vaccination on a long-term basis, and an exit strategy should be defined on the basis of regular reviews of the disease situation;
- that access to poultry can be difficult in dispersed backyard and smallholder farming systems;
- the need for transparency in the use of vaccination, information about the effectiveness of vaccination campaigns and virus circulation after vaccination and sharing of field data;
- the need to prevent unjustified trade barriers associated with vaccination;
- the need to preserve and protect valuable birds, such as certain poultry breeds (conservation of genetic biodiversity), zoo birds, pet birds, ornamental birds and (grand) parent flocks;
- that there are no indications of negative effects on human health associated with vaccination of poultry or consumption of their products;
- the need for high-quality veterinary services to implement and monitor vaccination strategies and all other preventive measures and control programmes, including early detection and response;
- the need to involve the public and private sectors together with veterinary services for successful prevention and control of HPAI;
- that the sustainability of vaccination strategies requires private and public commitment and cost sharing;
- the need for good veterinary governance, strong political commitment and appropriate legislation; and
- the need for appropriate communication and awareness of the risks for avian influenza of both poultry and humans as part of vaccination campaigns:

RECOMMENDS:

1. implementation of the OIE standards, guidelines and recommendations, the FAO guidelines and recommendations and the FAO-OIE global strategy on HPAI;
2. that importing countries respect the OIE standards in order to avoid unjustified trade barriers associated with vaccination against avian influenza;
3. adoption of an iterative approach to disease prevention and control, involving continuous assessment of the disease situation due to HPAI and the success of prevention and control strategies, so as to be able to modify or adjust the strategies as needed;
4. that the objectives of any vaccination strategy be defined before implementation in a country or region;

5. that use of vaccination, when relevant, be considered an addition to classical methods, such as stamping-out and increased biosecurity, but always in combination with the classical methods;
6. that vaccination be considered a valuable approach for reducing infection in endemic situations and that such countries be considered high priorities for preventive blanket vaccination programmes;
7. that vaccination be considered on the basis of a comprehensive analysis, including risk assessment of the country situation and context, covering:
   - the disease situation in the country (e.g. endemicity, number and location of outbreaks);
   - consideration of preventive blanket vaccination to control the virus in endemically infected countries;
   - the structure of poultry production sectors 1-4, the market chain and poultry density;
   - the risks for introduction and subsequent secondary spread;
   - the expected costs and benefits of vaccination to various stakeholders, taking into account impacts on consumption in rural and urban areas, and production and trade in different farming systems;
   - the feasibility, constraints and costs of using vaccination in comparison or in combination with other methods;
   - the availability and quality of veterinary diagnostic laboratories;
   - the quality of the veterinary services and the institutional environment;
   - the capability of animal health systems to implement various prevention and control measures, including vaccination;
   - the availability of quality-controlled vaccine authorized according to local regulatory standards;
   - the possible impact on consumer behaviour (fears about food safety) and subsequent market price changes; and
   - appropriation of policies by stakeholders, including poultry owners;
8. that a decision support method be designed for policy-makers, which should be incorporated into national preparedness plans on the basis of the criteria listed in operative paragraph 7;
9. that vaccination plans be an integral part of contingency and emergency preparedness plans;
10. adoption of a comprehensive approach, combining tools and measures for HPAI prevention, containment and elimination, in countries and subregions;
11. that any vaccination policy include an exit strategy for termination of vaccination, after reconsideration of the prevailing conditions at regional and national level;
12. that countries consider the use of vaccination to protect valuable birds, such as certain poultry breeds (conservation of germ plasm genetic biodiversity), zoo birds, pet birds, ornamental birds, (grand)parent flocks and fighting cocks, when there is an increased risk for infection;

13. that vaccination plans specifically address the issue of vaccination in smallholder and backyard farming systems, where high-level vaccine coverage is difficult to achieve (participatory, community-based approaches supervised by veterinary authorities could be integrated into the vaccination plan);
14. that countries ensure the availability of sufficient quality-controlled vaccine in their contingency plans, when necessary by establishing vaccine banks, strategic stockpiling of vaccines or arrangements with vaccine producers;
15. that countries design all accompanying measures, methods and protocols for post-vaccination monitoring, comprising:
    - evaluations of immunity;
    - monitoring of the circulation of field virus in vaccinated flocks;
    - routine testing of dead birds on farms;
    - clinical examination and monitoring of live-bird markets; and
    - monitoring of the genetic and antigenic characteristics of the circulating field virus;
16. that countries set up appropriate capacity-building programmes, including training in epidemiology, disease surveillance and reporting, field and laboratory diagnosis, vaccination skills, campaign implementation, farming system guidance, socioeconomic analysis, programme evaluation, decision-making and policy-making;
17. that countries enact the appropriate legislation and governance to implement HPAI control measures, including vaccination, and the means to enforce it and to streamline vaccine authorization;
18. evaluation and strengthening of veterinary services and public-private partnerships, including farmers' organizations;
19. promotion of cost-sharing for public and private goods and advocacy for investments by governments and the international community to ensure the sustainability of intervention strategies;
20. that commercial poultry establishments reinforce their engagement in the control of HPAI with national authorities;
21. increased investment in production of high-quality vaccines through private initiatives with local partnerships and increased availability of vaccines, particularly in developing countries;
22. the establishment and funding of research programmes in the following fields:
    - the epidemiology of avian influenza viruses, including molecular epidemiology and the role of wild birds and other animal species;
    - decision support models that take into account all relevant factors;
    - the onset, level and duration of immunity after vaccination in various species under laboratory and field conditions and immunosuppressive factors that might interfere with the development of immunity;
    - combination of avian influenza vaccination with control of other poultry diseases, particularly Newcastle disease;

- development of new and improved vaccines and accompanying diagnostic tests, and definition of the requirements for high-quality vaccines;
- establishment of antigen banks;
- optimal methods for surveillance;
- possible social and economic impacts of vaccination, including on production, consumption and trade, in comparison with other control methods;
- cost-effective methods of administration (one shot) and delivery, particularly for smallholder and backyard systems (participatory approaches, private sector delivery);
- epidemiological and economical analysis of data collected during vaccination campaigns; and
- stakeholder alliances with OFFLU and platforms like the European Technology Platform for Global Animal Health to coordinate global research on avian influenza;

23. that published and presented information on vaccination against avian influenza be evaluated and summarized in a peer-reviewed publication;
24. the design of communication strategies to enhance vaccine coverage, mitigate possible market impacts and clarify consumer concerns about food safety and the concerns of farming communities; and
25. recognition that control of HPAI, including by vaccination, has a substantial component of global public good and that the international community should continue to support control, particularly in developing countries.

List of Participants

••••••••••••••••••

ALDERS Robyn, FAO Regional Office, 39 Phra Atit Road, Bangkok 10200 Thailand, robyn.alders@gmail.com

ABD EL-AZIZ Saber, IFT St. no. 9, Block 6103, Mokattam Cairo 11439, Egypt, technical@ift-online.com

ABOLNIK Celia, ARC-Onderstepoort Veterinary Institute, Old Soutpan Road, Onderstepoort, Pretoria 0110, South Africa, abolnikc@arc.agric.za

ADAM YAGOUB Ismail, Ministry of Animal Resources of the Republic of the Sudan c/o Sudan Embassy Via Prati della Farnesina, 57 Rome 00194, Italy, permrepoffice_sudanembassyrome@yahoo.it

AL BURAIKAN Yousef, Dept of Animal Health, Public Authority for Agriculture Affairs and Fish Resources (PAAF), PO Box 21422 Safat, Kuwait 13075, Kuwait, animhlth@paaf.gov.ku

AL MULLA Farida, Public Authority for Agriculture Affairs & Fish Resources (PAAF), PO Box 21422, Safat Kuwait 13075, Kuwait, animhlth@paaf.gov.ku, f_molla@hotmail.com

AL SUMAIT Abdullah, Public Authority for Agriculture Affairs & Fish Resources (PAAF) PO Box 21422, Kuwait 13075, Kuwait, animhlth@paaf.gov.kw

ALBA CASALS Anna, Campus de Bellaterra, Edifici V Bellaterra, Barcelona, 08193, Spain, ana.alba@cresa.uab.es

ALBISHER Abdullah, Ministry of Agriculture, Department of Animals Resources, King Abdulaziz Street, Riyadh 11195, Saudi Arabia, aalbisher@yahoo.com

ALDERS Robyn, International Rural Poultry Centre, Kyeema Foundation, G.P.O. Box 3023, Brisbane 4001, Australia, robyna@kyeemafoundation.org and robyn.alders@gmail.com

ALI Bahman Hassan, Ministry of Agricultur Kurdistan Region, Nishtiman Q. Erbil, 066, Iraq, bahman_hassan@yahoo.com

ALI Hussein, IFT St. no. 9, Block 6103, Mokattam Cairo 11439, Egypt, technical@ift-online.com

ALI AHMED AL-MOMANIL Ziad, Ministry of Agriculture Amman Amman, Jordan 2099, Jordan, zmomany@yahoo.com

AL-MUBARAK Majdi, Ministry oF Agriculture Jordan, Salt 320, Jordan, agri@moa.gov.jo

ALY Mona, Central Laboratory for veterinary Quality Control on Poultry Production Nadi Elseid – Dokki, V Giza 246, Egypt, monaaly4@hotmail.com

AMANFU William, UN - FAO Sudan Embassy, Via Prati della Farnesina, 57 Rome 00194, Italy, william.amanfu@fao.org

AMARAL Cristina, FAO Viale delle Terme di Caracalla Roma, 00153, Italy, cristina.amaral@fao.org

AMOREK-SALAMONOWICZ Elzbieta, National Veterinary Resaearch Institute, AL. Partyzantow 57 Pulawy 24-100, Poland, elsam@piwet.pulawy.pl

ANDREASEN Claire, Iowa State University, College of Veterinary Medicine, Ames, Iowa 50011, USA, candreas@iastate.edu

ANNELLI Joseph, USDA/APHIS 1400 Independence Ave. SW, Room S-310, South Building Stop 9820,Washington, DC 20250, USA, joseph.f.annelli@aphis.usda.gov

ARRIOLA Jose Manuel, Bachoco, Av. Norte 11 Equina Poniente 4, Ciudad Industrial Celaya, Guanajuato, 38010, Mexico, jose.arriola@bachoco.net

ASKAROGLU Haluk, Ministry of Agriculture, General Directorate of Protection Control, Akay Caddesi, No. 3 Bakanliklar, Ankara 06100, Turkey, haluka@kkgm.gov.tr

BALDINELLI Francesca, Istituto Superiore di Sanità Viale Regina Elena 299, Rome, 00161, Italy, francescabaldinelli@libero.it

BANDLI Risch, Institute of Veterinary Bacteriology/ NRGK, Vetsuisse Faculty, University of Zurich, Winterthurerstrasse 270, Zürich 8057, Switzerland, risch@bandli.net

BANKS Jill, Veterinary Laboratories Agency, Woodham Lane, Addlestone, Surrey KT15 3NB, United Kingdom, j.banks@vla.defra.gsi.gov.uk

BANO Luca, Istituto Zooprofilattico delle Venezie viale Brigata Treviso 13/a Treviso, 30100, Italy, lbano@izsvenezie.it

BARBUS Mihaela, Permanent Representation of Romania to the EU, rue Montoyer Brussels 1000, Belgium, mihaela.barbus@rpro.eu

BARTELING Simon, Simbar Consultancy, Nieuwe Keizersgracht 438, Amsterdam 1018VG, Netherlands, simbar@planet.nl

BAR-YAACOV Keren, Norwegian Food Safety Authority, PO Box 383, Brumunddal N-2381, Norway, kebay@mattilsynet.no

BASHIR Taha Mohamed, Ministry of Animal Resources of the Republic of the Sudan c/o Sudan Embassy, Via Prati della Farnesina 57, Rome 00194, Italy, permrepoffice_sudanembassyrome@yahoo.it

BEATO Maria Serena, IZSVe, Viale dell' Università 10 Legnaro, Padua, 35020, Italy, msbeato@izsvenezie.it

BEDARD Brian, World Bank, 1818 H street NW, Washington DC 20433, USA, bbedard@worldbank.org

BEERS Peter, Department of Agriculture and Fisheries, Edmund Barton Building, Act G Po Box 858, Canberra, Australia, peter.beers@daff.gov.au

BELL Jonathan, USAID Community Based Avian Influenza Control Gedung BRI II, Suite 2807 J. Jend. Sudirman, Jakarta, Indonseia, jonathan_bell@dai.com

BEN JEBARA Karim, OIE, 12 rue de Prony 75017 Paris, France, k.benjebara@oi.int

BENICASA Tamara, OIE, 12 rue de Prony, 75017 Paris, France, pub.sales@oie.int

BENSABER Amina, Seppic Tour Kupka C 7 Boulevard Frank Kupka, Paris La Défense Cedex 92039, France, amina.bensaber@airliquide.com

BERBARI Nagib, Ministry of Agriculture, Bir Hassan Beirut, BP 40010 Baabda, Lebanon, nberberi@hotmail.com

BERGAMINI Paolo, AUSL 22 Regione Veneto Via Ospedale 5, Villafranca di Verona 37069, Italy, dvetisola@ulss22.ven.it

BERHANE Yohannes, Canadian Food Inspection Agency/NCFAD, 1015 Arlington Street, Winnipeg/Manitoba, R3E 3M4, Canada, BerhaneY@inspection.gc.ca

BERTRAND François, Seppic Tour Kupka C, 7 Boulevard Frank Kupka, Paris La Défense Cedex 92039, France, francois.bertrand@airliquide.com

BESSI Olivia, Ministry oh Health, Piazza Marconi 25, Rome 00144, Italy, o.bessi@sanita.it

BIARNES Mar, CESAC Carretera Castellvell, s/n Reus, 43206, Spain, mbiarnes@cesac.org

BIRES Jozef, State Veterinary and Food Administration of the Slovak Republic, Botanicka st. 17, Bratislava 842 13, Slovakia, bires@svssr.sk

BISSCHOP Shahn, Poultry Reference Centre, Faculty of Veterinary Science, University of Pretoria, Private Bag X04, Onderstepoort Pretoria, 0181, South Africa, shahn.bisschop@up.ac.za

BISWAS Dipankar, Kopar Khairane, Sector 11 PO: Kopar Khairane, Navi, Mumbay, 400 709, India, dipankarbiswas2001@yahoo.co.in

BONFANTI Lebana, Istituto Zooprofilattico delle Venezie, Viale dell'Università, 10 Legnaro (PD) 35020, Italy, lbonfanti@izsvenezie.it

BORISOV Vladimir, FGI 600901, Yur'evets, Vladimir, Russia Vladimir, 600901, Russia, gonova@arriah.ru

BOWES Victoria, British Columbia Ministry of Agriculture, Animal Health Centre, 1767 Angus Campbell Rd, Abbotsford, V3G 2M3, Canada, Victoria.Bowes@gov.bc.ca

BRANCHETTI Mauro, AUSL di Reggio Emilia, Via A. Catalani 16, Reggio Emilia, 42100, Italy, branchettim@ausl.re.it / brank2@libero.it

BRICHESE Michele, Veneto Region Dorsoduro 3493, Venezia 30125, Italy, michele.brichese@regione.veneto.it

BRIOUDES Aurelie, FAO 3 Nguyen Gia Thieu, Hanoi, PO BOX 63, Vietnam, aurelie@fao.org.vn

BRONZATO Giulano, ASL 21 Legnago, Via C. Giannella 1, Legnago Verona 37045, Italy, veterinaria.leg@aulsslegnago.it

BROWN Ian, FAO/OIE/EU Reference Laboratory for AI Veterinary Laboratories Agency Weybridge, New Haw, Addlestone, Surrey KT15 3NB, United Kingdom, i.h.brown@vla.defra.gsi.gov.uk

BRÜCKNER Gideon, OIE, 12 rue de Prony 75017 Paris, France, g.bruckner@oie.int

BRUSCHKE Christiane, OIE, 12 rue de Prony 75017 Paris, France, c.bruschke@oie.int

BU Zhigao, Harbin Veterinary Research Institute, 427 Maduan Street, Harbin 150001, China, zgbu@yahoo.com

BUBLOT Michael, Merial, 254 rue Marcel Merieux Lyon 69007, France, michel.bublot@merial.com

BULLIDO Rosario, Spanish Agency of Medicines and Medical Devices, Parque Empresarial Las Mercedes. C/ Campezo 1, Edificio 8. Madrid 28022, Spain, rbullido@agemed.es

BUSANI Luca, Istituto Zooprofilattico Sperimentale delle Venezie, Viale dell'Università 10 Legnaro, Padua, 35020, Italy, crev.lbusani@izsvenezie.it

BUSSIONI Yasser, General Organization for Veterinary Services 1, Nady El-said Street, Dokki, Giza 12311, Egypt, tawfik@claes.sci.eg

CAPUA Ilaria, Istituto Zooprofilattico Sperimentale delle Venezie, Viale dell'Università 10 Legnaro, Padua, 35020, Italy, icapua@izsvenezie.it

CARDENAS Leonides, USDA/APHIS, 120-122 Wireless Rd., Bangkok, 10330, Thailand, ned.l.cardenas@aphis.usda.gov

CARLSSON Ulla, Statens Veterinärmedicinska Anstalt Uppsala, Uppsala SE-751 89, Sweden, ulla.carlsson@sva.se

CATBAGAN Davinio, Bureau of Animal Industry, Visayas Avenue, Diliman Quezon City 1100, Philippines, dir.bai@manilaonline.com

CATTOLI Giovanni, Istituto Zooprofilattico Sperimentale delle Venezie Adresse : viale dell'Università 10, Legnaro Padova 35020, Italy, mmandelli@izsvenezie.it

CAYA François, Canadian Food Inspection Agency, 59 Camelot Drive, Ottawa, Ontario K1A 0Y9, Canada, cayaf@inspection.gc.ca

CAZABAN Christophe, CEVA Santé Animale, 159 avenue Georges Pomidou, BP 126, Libourne CEDEX, 33501, France, christophe.cazaban@ceva.com

CECCHINATO Mattia, Medicine Faculty, University of Padua, Viale dell'Università, 16, Agripolis Legnaro (PD,) 35020, Italy, mattia.cecchinato@unipd.it

CELESTINI Corrado, USL 7 Ragusa, Ronco Salice 2 noto, 96017, Italy, corradocelestini@supereva.it

CEOLIN Chiara, University of Padova, viale dell 'Università, Agripolis Padova, 35020 Legnaro, Italy, chiara.ceolin@unipd.it c.ceolin@libero.it

CHAISINGH Arunee, National Institute of Animal Health, Chatuchak, Bangkok 10900, Thailand, naih8@dld.go.th

CHAITAWEESUB Prasit, Department of Livestock Development, 69/1 Phyathai Road, Bangkok, 10400, Thailand, dcontrol1@dld.go.th

CHANG Siow Foong, Agri-Food and Veterinary Authority of Singapore, Veterinary Public Health Centre, 10 Perahu Road, 718837, Singapore, chang_siow_foong@ava.gov.sg

CHANOCH Yuvel, 33 Hanadiv St, Herzeliya 46100, Israel, rhyorama@gmail.com

CHERIF Aoumeur, Boehringer Ingelheim Vetmedica, S.A. de C.V., Calle 30 No. 2614, Zona Industrial, Guadalajara, Jalisco 44940, Mexico, cherif_vet@yahoo.fr

CILLONI Filippo, Istituto Zooprofilattico Sperimentale delle Venezie, Viale dell'Università 10 Legnaro, Padua, 35020, Italy, fcilloni@izsvenezie.it

CLAASSEN Ivo, Central Institute for Infectious Diseases, PO BOX 2004, Lelystad 8203 AA, Netherlands, ivo.claassen@wur.nl

CLARK James, Canadian Food Inspection Agency, 59 Camelot Drive, Ottawa, Ontario K1A 0Y9, Canada, clarkj@inspection.gc.ca

CLARK Alice, RSPCA, Wilberforce Way Southwater, Horsham RH13 9RS, United Kingdom, aclark@rspca.org.uk

CLERKIN Patrick, Avian Influenza Action Group, US Department of State 1800 G Street, NW, Room 2321A, Washington, DC 20560, USA, clerkinpj@state.gov

COATS Max, USDA-FAS American Embassy Jakarta Unit 8129 (AGR) FPO AP, 96520-8129, USA, mcoats@earth-comm.com

COLE Kimberly, University of Arkansas, POSC O-114, 1260 W. Maple Street, Fayetteville, Arkansas, 72701, USA, kimcole@uark.edu

COLLINS Lisa, Compassion in World Farming, River Court Mill Lane Godalming, Surrey, GU7 1EZ, United Kingdom, lisa@ciwf.co.uk,

COVEN Fethiye, The Misnistry of Agriculture and Rural Affairs, Osman Kibar Meydan&#305, Ege Universitesi Kavsagı ZMIR 35010, Turkey, covenfethiye@yahoo.com

CRISTALLI Alessandro, Istituto Zooprofilattico Sperimentale delle Venezie, Viale dell'Università 10 Legnaro, Padua 35020, Italy, acristalli@izsvenezie.it

CUI Czifra, The National Veterinary Institute, Travvägen 20, Uppsala SE-75 189, Sweden, gyorgy.czifra@sva.se

DALLA POZZA Giuseppe, Istituto Zooprofilattico Sperimentale delle Venezie, Viale dell'Università 10 Legnaro, Padua 35020, Italy, asartor@izsvenezie.it

DALLA POZZA Manuela, Istituto Zooprofilattico Sperimentale delle Venezie, Viale dell'Università 10 Legnaro, Padua 35020, Italy, crev.mdallapozza@izsvenezie.it

DANIELS Peter, CSIRO Livestock Industries, Private Bag 24, Geelong, VIC 3220, Australia, peter.daniels@csiro.au

DANRONGWATANAPOKIN Sudarat, USAID 3rd Floor, GPF Witthayu Tower A 93/1 Wireless Road Lumpini, Bangkok 10330, Thailand, sdamrongwatanapokin@usaid.gov

DAUPHINE Gwenaëlle, FAO, Viale delle Terme di Caracalla, Rome 00153, Italy, gwenaelle.dauphin@fao.org

DAVID Bruce, National Veterinary Institute of Norway, Postboks 8156 Dep. Oslo N-0033, Norway, bruce.david@vetinst.no

DE KLERK Fred, Food and Consumer Product Safety Authority, PO Box 19506, The Hague 2500 CM, Netherlands, fred.de.klerk@vwa.nl

DE LA ROCQUE Stephane, FAO Viale delle Terme di Caracalla Roma, 00153, Italy, stephane.delarocque@fao.org

DE RUI Stefano, AZ. ULSS, 8 Asolo via San Rocco 68, Segusino 31040, Italy, derui@ulssasolo.ven.it

DE WIT Jacobus, Animal Health Service GD Deventer, Arnsbergstraat 7, Deventer 7400 AA, Netherlands, j.d.wit@gddeventer.com

DELLA VALENTINA Marcos, AMADORI Via Bonfadina 9, Cazzago S. Martino, 25046, Italy, marco.dellavalentina@amadori.it

DETOLLA Louis, University of Maryland School of Medicine, 10 South Pine St., MSTF, Room G-100, Baltimore, MD 21201-1192, USA, detolla@vetmed.umaryland.edu

DEVILLE Sebastian, Seppic Tour Kupka C.7, Boulevard Frank Kupka, Paris La Défense Cedex 92039, France, sebastien.deville@airliquide.com

DI MODUGNO Girolamo, Facoltà Veterinaria, Strada Prov. Casdamassima Km 3 Valenzano Bari 70010, Italy, g.dimodugno@veterinaria.uniba .it

DODOVSKI Aleksandar, Faculty of Veterinary Medicine, Skopje, ul. Lazar PopTrajkov 5-7 Skopje 1000, Macedonia, adodovski@fvm.ukim.edu.mk

DOMENECH Joseph, FAO, Viale delle Terme di Caracalla Roma, 00153, Italy, joseph.domenech@fao.org

DUCATEZ Mariette, Institute of Immunology, National Public Health Laboratory, 20A rue Auguste Lumière, Luxembourg L-1950, Luxembourg, Mariette.Ducatez@lns.etat.lu

DUNDON William, Istituto Zooprofilattico Sperimentale delle Venezie, Viale dell'Università 10 Legnaro, Padua 35020, Italy, wdundon@izsvenezie.it

EK-KOMMONEN Christine, Finnish Food Safety Authority Mustialankatu 3, Helsinki, 00790, Finland, christine.ek-kommonen@evira.fi

ELHADY Mohamed, IFT St. no. 9, Block 6103, Mokattam, Cairo 11439, Egypt, technical@ift-online.com

ELKADY Magdy, IFT st. no. 9, block 6103, Cairo 11439, Egypt, technical@ift-online.com

ELKIN Nathan, BIOVAC PO Box 300 Orakiva, 30 600, Israel, elkin@poultrymed.com

ELSKEN Lawrence, Department of Agriculture, Center for Veterinary Biologics, 510 S. 17th Street, Suite 104, Ames, Iowa, 50010 USA, lawrence.a.elsken@aphis.usda.gov

ELTAYEB ELFAKI Mohamed, UN, FAO Sudan Embassy, Via Prati della Farnesina 57, Rome 00194, Italy, permrepoffice_sudanembassyrome@yahoo.it

ESCHER Martina, Università degli Studi di Perugia/ Istituto Superiore di Sanità Viale Regina Elena, 299 Rome, 00161, Italy, martina.escher@iss.it

ESPINOZA Cora, Servicio Nacional de Sanidad y Calidad Agroaliementaria, Paseo Colon 367 4to piso, Ciudad de Buenos Aires 1063, Argentina, avesygranja@senasa.gov.ar

ESPOSITO Roberto, European Commission, POBox 782890, Sandton Johannesburg 2146, South Africa, roberto@casamatteo.net

ESPUNYA Enric, HIPRA Av. La Selva, 135 Amer Girona 17170, Spain, eem@hipra.com

FAVERO Laura, Veneto Region Dorsoduro 3493, Venezia 30125, Italy, laura.favero@regione.veneto.it

FERNANDEZ Lorena, TRAGSEGA c/Maldonado, 58, Madrid 28006, Spain, lfernan2@tragsa.es

FINLEY Melissa, Sandia National Laboratories PO Box 5800, Mail Stop 1371 Albuquerque, New Mexico 87104, USA, mfinley@sandia.gov

FRENCH Cheryl, USDA-APHIS International Services 2130 Dakar Place Dulles, Virginia 20189, USA, cheryl.m.french@aphis.usda.gov

FROLOV Sergey, FGI ARRIAH - 600901, Russia, Vladimir, Yur'evets, 600901, Russia, gonova@arriah.ru

GAGLIARDI Stefano, Con.Av. Via Punta di Ferro, 2 Piazzale Foro Boario, Forlì, 47100, Italy, aerac@agraria.it

GARCIA Emilio, Ministerio de la Agricultura Pesca y Alimentacion C/ Alfonso XII, 62, Madrid 28014, Spain, egarciam@mapya.es

GHIGGIA Stefania, Istituto zooprofilattico P.L.V., V.Villa della regina 12, Torino 10131, Italy, ghiggia.s@libero.it

GHINATO Carlo, Ser. vet. Emilia Romagna Regione, Via Aldo Moro n-30, Bologna 40013, Italy, viabon@ libero.it

GILBERT Jeffrey, FAO, 3 Nguyen Gia Thieu, Hanoi N/A, Vietnam, jeffrey.Gilbert@fao.org

GIROLAMO Di Modungo, Dipartimento Sanità Benessere animale, Università Studi, Facoltà Veterinaria, Strada Prov. Casdamassima Km 3, Valenzano (Bari), 70010, Italy, g.dimodugno@veterinaria.uniba .it

GONZALEZ Carlos, Boehringer Ingelheim Vetmedica, Calle 30, No. 2614, Zona Industrial, Guadalajara, Jalisco, 44940, Mexico, carlos.gonzalez@gua.boehringer-ingelheim.com

GOUJGOULOVA Gabriela, NDRVMI,190 Lomsko shose Blvd,Sofia, C.P.1231, Bulgaria, gvgoujgoulova@bav.bg

GRAHAM Robert, Development Alternatives, Inc. (DAI), 7600 Wisconsin Avenue, Suite 200, Bethesda, MD 20814, USA, ross_graham@dai.com

GRASSELLI Aldo, SIVEMP, Via nizza 11 Roma, 00198, Italy, segrenaz@sivemp.it

GUBERTI Vittorio, Istituto Nazionale Fauna Selvatica, Via Ca' Fornacetta 9, Ozzano E. 40064, Italy, vittorio.guberti@infs.it

HALL Sara, CFSPH 2160 Vet Med ISU, Ames, IA, 50011, USA, lhurley@iastate.edu

HALL Cheryl, USDA/APHIS 120-122 Wireless Rd, Bangkok 10330, Thailand, cheryl.i.hall@aphis.usda.gov

HAMILTON Keith, Defra, 1a Page Street, London SW1P 4PQ, United Kingdom, keith.hamilton@defra.gsi.gov.uk

HANSEN Hane, Danish Veterinary and Food Administration, Moerkhoej Bygade 19, Soeborg 2860, Denmark, hmh@fvst.dk

HARI Aleksandra, Veterinary Administation of the Republic of Slovenia Parmova, 53 Ljubljana 1000, Slovenia, aleksandra.hari@gov.si

HASSAN Salah Mahdi, College of Veterinary Medicine, University of Dohuk, Dohuk, 062, Iraq, alhashemi2004@yahoo.com

HASSAN Magdy, IFT - Mokattam, Cairo, 11439, Egypt, technical@ift-online.com

HERNANDEZ Rolando, Hannover Re-Karl-Wiechert-Allee 50 Hannover, 30625, Germany, patricia.becker@hannover-re.com

HERRMANN Andreas, Merial, 29, avenue Tony Garnier, BP 7123, Lyon, 69348 Cedex 07, France, andreas.herrmann@merial.com

HIBRAHIMA Diakite, Ministère de la Santé Publique, Boulevard du Commerce, Conarky 6003, Republique de Guinee, popuenviron20052010@yahoo.fr

HOEL Kristian, P.O. Box 218 Økern, Oslo 0510, Norway, kristian.hoel@fjorfe.org

HORNICKOVA Jitka, State Veterinary Institute Prague, Sidlistni 24, Praha 6 Lysolaje, Prague 165 03, Czech Republic, jitka.hornickova@svupraha.cz

HOSNY Farid, IFT - Mokattam, Cairo, 11439, Egypt, technical@ift-online.com

HUIBERT Maurice, Ministry of Agriculture, Nature and Food Quality Bezuidenhoutseweg 73 Den Haag, 2500 EK, Netherlands, h.maurice@minlnv.nl

HUSSEIN Ali, IFT St. no. 9, Block 6103, Mokattam, Cairo 11439, Egypt, technical@ift-online.com

HUTCHINGS Donna, Canadian Food Inspection Agency 2 Constellation Crescent, Ottawa, Ontario K1A 0Y9, Canada, hutchingsd@inspection.gc.ca

IL IDRISSI Ahmed, UN-FAO Sudan Embassy, Via Prati della Farnesina, 57 Rome 00194, Italy, ahmed.elidrissi@fao.org

IRZA Victor, FGI ARRIAH - 600901, Russia, Vladimir, Yur'evets Vladimir, 600901, Russia, gonova@arriah.ru

ISBENTCHIAN Hagop, Laboratorio Avimex, Maíz No. 18, Colonia Granjas Esmeralda, Iztapalapa, Mexico City, 09810, Mexico, hisbent@worldnet.att.net

JAGT Erik, Intervet International BV, Wim de Korverstraat 35, 5830AA Boxmeer, Netherlands, erik.jagt@intervet.com

JONES Andrew, Department for Environment, Food and Rural Affairs, Area 605, 1A Page Street, London, SW1P 4PQ, United Kingdom, andrew.jones@defra.gsi.gov.uk

JONES Peter, International Federation for Animal Health (IFAM) 1, rue Defacaz B-1000, Brussels, Belgium, p.jones@ifahsec.org

JORGENSEN Poul Henrik, Danish Veterinary Institute, Hangoevej 2, Aarhus N 8200, Denmark, phj@dfvf.dk

KAHN Sarah, OIE, 12 rue de Prony, 75017 Paris, France, s.kahn@oie.int

KAKEL Dieyar, Boehringer Ingelheim Pharma Business Gulf States, P.O.Box 3264 Dubai, United Arab Emirates, dieyar@dxb.boehringer-ingelheim.com

KALPRAVIDH Wantanee, FAO Regional Office For Asia and The Pacific, 39 Maliwan Mansion, PHRA Atit Road, Bangkok 10200, Thailand, wantanee.kalpravidh@fao.org

KAMARUDIN Isa, Ministry of Agriculture and Agro-based Industry, Level 5, Block Podium, Lot 4G1, Presint 4, Putrajaya62630, Kuala Lumpur 62630, Malaysia, kamar57@yahoo.com

KANGA Kouame, Direction des Services Vétérinaires, BP 88 Abidjan, Ivory Coast, kceml@yahoo.fr

KAPUR Shashi, Poultry Federation of India 225, Sector 14 Gurgaon, Haryana 122001, India, kapur01@gmail.com

KHAFAGA RHAMAN Abdel, IFT St. no. 9, Block 6103, Mokattam Cairo, 11439, Egypt, technical@ift-online.com

KHALIFA Mohamed, Central Laboratory for Veterinary Quality Control on Poultry Production (CLQP), Nadi El Said Street, Dokki Cairo 11231, Egypt, shereengalal@yahoo.com

KIDA Hiroshi, School of veterinary Medicine and Research Center for Zoonosis Control, Hokkaido University, Kita-18, Nishi-9, Kitaku, Sapporo 060-0818, Japan, kida@vetmed.hokudai.ac.jp

KIM Chang-Seob, Ministry of Agriculture and Forestry #1, Joong-Ang, Kwa-Cheon Kyunggi-do 427-760, Korea, cvo@maf.go.kr, cskim@maf.go.kr

KIM Yong Joo, Avian Disease Division, National Veterinary Research and Quarantine Service 480 Anyang 6 dong, An Yang City Gyeonggi-do 430-824, Korea, kimyj@nvrqs.go.kr, kyjvet@yahoo.com

KIVIRUUSU Sirpa, Finnish Food Safety Authority Evira Mustialankatu 3 Helsinki, 00790, Finland, sirpa.kiviruusu@evira.fi

KOCH Guus, Central Institute for Animal Disease Control Lelystad (CIDC-Lelystad) Department of Virology D, Post-box 2004 8203 AA Lelystad, Netherlands, Guus.Koch@WUR.NL

KRIZ Nicolaus, European Medicines Agency, 7 Westferry Circus, Canary Wharf London E14 4HB, United Kingdom, Nikolaus.Kriz@emea.europa.eu

LADDOMADA Alberto, DG SANCO, European Commission, Rue Froissart 101, room 3/56, Brussels 1040, Belgium, alberto.laddomada@ec.europa.eu

LAMBERGA Kristine, Food and Veterinary Service of the Republic of Latvia, Repulikas laukums 2, Riga LV-1010, Lativia, kristine.lamberga@pvd.gov.lv

LAMSENS Gerard, SPF Santé Publique, Sécurité de la Chaîne Alimentaire et Environnement, Eurostation II, 7e étage, Place Victor Horta 40, bte 10, Bruxelles 1060, Belgium, gerard.lamsens@health.fgov.be

LANY Peter, University of Veterinary and Pharmaceutical Sciences, Brno Palackeho 1/3, Brno 612 42, Czech Republic, lanyp@vfu.cz

LAZAR Niculae, National Sanitary Veterinary and Food Safety Authority Negusteori Street n°1 bis, Bucharest 023951, Romania, lazar@ansv.ro

LEBOUCQ Nadege, World Bank, 1818 H street NW, Washington DC 20433, USA, nleboucq@worldbank.org

LECH Ewa, General Veterinary Inspectorate, ul. Wspolna 30, Warsaw 00-930, Poland, ewa.lech@wetgiw.gov.pl

LEFORBAN Yves, Ministère de l'Agriculture et de la Pêche, 251 rue de Vaugirard, Paris 75015, France, yves.leforban@agriculture.gouv.fr

LEKCHAROENSUK Porntippa, Faculty of Veterinary Medicine, Kasetsart University, 50 Paholyothin Rd, Chatuchak Bangkok 10900, Thailand, fvetptn@ku.ac.th

LEOWIJUK Chaweewan, Department of Livestock Development, 69/1 Phayathai Road, Ratchatawee Bangkok 10400, Thailand, chaweewl@dld.go.th

LESCEU Stéphanie, ID VET 167 Rue Medhi BenBarka, Zone Garosud, Montpellier 34070, France, stephanie.lesceu@id-vet.com

LIVEN Eivind, Norwegian Food Safety Authority, Mattilsynet Mattilsynet, Felles Postmottak Postboks 383 Oslo, 2381 Brumunddal, Norway, eivind.liven@mattilsynet.no

LOGAN-HENFREY Linda, USDA-APHIS-IS, 8 Kamali el Din Salah Garden City, 3000, Egypt, linda.l.logan@aphis.usda.gov

LONKOFF Ghislaine, Seppic, Tour Kupka C, 7 Boulevard Frank Kupka, Paris La Defense Cedex 92039, France, laurent.dupuis@airliquide.com

LOVELL Kevin, Southern African Poultry Association, PO Box 1202 Honeydew, Gauteng 2040, South Africa, kevin@sapoultry.co.za

LOZANO Bernardo, Laboratorio Avimex, Maíz No. 18, Colonia Granjas Esmeralda, Delegación Iztapalapa, Mexico City 09810, Mexico, lozano@avimex.com.mx

LUBROTH Juan, FAO, Viale delle Terme di Caracalla Roma, 00153, Italy, Juan.Lubroth@fao.org

LUCIO Eduardo, Investigación Aplicada, 7 Norte 416, Col. Centro, Tehuacán, Puebla 75700, Mexico, elucio@grupoidisa.com

MACGREGOR-SKINNER Gavin, USDA, 1300 Pennsylvania Avenue, NW, GH/HIDN/ID, Rm 5.9-B Washington DC, 20523, USA, gmacgregor-skinner@usaid.gov

MAFFEO Angela, ASLCE 2 -24,via mario gelosoruviano, 81010, Caserta -Campania, Italy, epi.occupaslce2@virgilio.it

MAMODE Ismet, Food and Allied Indutries, Royal road Gentilly, Moka C.P. NIL, Mauritius, ism.mamode@failgroup.intnet.mu

MANDOLA Maria Lucia, IZVP, Liguria E Valle D'Aosta, Via Bologna 148, Torino 10154, Italy, marialucia.mandola@izsto.it

MANIN Timofey, FGI ARRIAH, 600901, Russia, Vladimir, Yur'evets, Vladimir, 600901, Russia, gonova@arriah.ru

MANSER Paul, Defra, 1A Page Street, London SW1P 4PQ, United Kingdom, paul.a.manser@defra.gsi.gov.uk

MANZAN Massimo, Az. ULSS 18 di Rovigo, Viale Tre Martiri n. 89, Rovigo 45100, Italy, veter.ro@azisanrovigo.it

MARABELLI Romano, Ministry of Health, Piazzale Marconi 25, Rome I-00144, Italy, alimentivet@sanità.it

MARANGON Stefano, Istituto Zooprofilattico delle Venezie Viale dell'Università, 10 Legnaro, Padua, 35020, Italy, dirsan@izsvenezie.it

MARINI Carla, Istituto Zooprofilattico Sperimentale Dell'Umbria e delle Marche, Via Gaetano Salvemini N. 1, Perugia, 06126, Italy, c.marini@izsum.it

MARTIN Jerry, Development Alternatives, Inc., 7600 Wisconsin Ave., Bethesda, MD 20814, USA, jerry_martin@dai.com

MCLEOD ANNI, FAO, Viale delle Terme di Caracalla, Roma 00100, Italy, Anni.McLeod@fao.org

MCATEER Billy, Department of Agriculture and Food, Agriculture House, Kildare Street, Dublin 2, Ireland, billy.mcateer@agriculture.gov.ie

MCCULLOUGH Kenneth, Institude of Virology and Immunoprophylaxis, Sensemattstrasse 293, Mittelhausern 3147, Switzerland, kenneth.mccullough@ivi.admin.ch

MEGGIOLARO Sergio, Aulss 22 Bussolengo, Via Ospedale 5, Villafranca di Verona 37069, Italy, smeggiolaro@ulss22.ven.it

MEHREZ Mona, IFT St. no. 9, Block 6103, Mokattam Cairo 11439, Egypt, technical@ift-online.com

MEINI Amelio, IntervetItalia, Via Walter Tobagi 7, Peschiera Borremeo (MI) 20068, Italy, amelio.meini@intervet.com

MELIOTA Francesco, FATRO S.P.A., Via Emilia 285, Ozzano dell'Emilia BO, 40064, Italy, biologici@fatro.it

MELLERGAARD Stig, Danish Veterinary and Food Administration, Mørkhøj Bygade 19, Søborg DK-2860, Denmark, stim@fvst.dk

METTENNLEITER Thomas, Friedrich-Loeffler-Institut, Boddenblick 5A, Greifswald-Insel Riems, 17493, Germany, thomas.mettenleiter@fli.bund.de

MICKLE Thomas, Merial 1112 Airport Parkway S.E., Gainesville, Georgia, 30506, USA, tom.mickle@merial.com

MINGUEZ-TUDELA ISABEL, EC SDME 8 8/96 Brussels 1049, Belgium, isabel.minguez-tudela@ec.europa.eu

MINTA Zenon, National Veterinary Research Institute, Al. Partyzantow 57, Pulawy 24-100, Poland, zminta@piwet.pulawy.pl

MOHAMMAD JAVAD Mehrabanpour, Istituto Zooprofilattico Sperimentale delle Venezie, Viale dell'Università 10 Legnaro, Padua 35020, Italy, mmandelli@izsvenezie.it

MOHAMMED Diyar Tayeb, Veterinary services and Animal Resources / Dohuk shahiden 1 - Shwat Road Dohuk 062, Iraq, diartayeb@yahoo.com

MOJZIS Miroslav, State Veterinary Institute, Pod Drahami 918, Zvolen, 96086 Slovakia, mojzis@svuzv.sk

MONPETIT Christiane, AFSSA 27, 31 avenue Général Leclerc, Maison Alfort 94700, France, c.monpetit@afssa,fr

MORENO Ana, IZS Lombardia ed Emilia Romagna, Via Bianchi 9, Brescia 25124, Italy, amoreno@bs.izs.it

MORIN Florence, AIDCO European Commission, 41 rue de la Loi, Bruxelles, Belgium 1000, florence.morin@ec.europa.eu

MORSTEIN Carola Von, GTZ GmbH, Dag-Haemmerskjoeld Weg 1-5, Eschborn, 65760 Germany, carola.morstein-von@gtz.de

MOTA Marcelo, Brazilian Ministry of Agriculture, Livestock and Food Supply, Esplanada dos Ministérios, Bloco D, Anexo A, sala 318. Brasília - DF. CEP. 70.043-900, Brazil, marcelomota@agricultura.gov.br

MUKARKER Imad, MoA- PA Ministry of Agriculture, Ramallah, Palestine, PO Box 197, Palestina, drimad_s@yahoo.com

MUNOZ Beatriz, Ministerio de la Agricultura Pesca y Alimentacion, C/ Alfonso XII, 62, Madrid 28014, Spain, bmunozhu@mapya.es

MUSAA Joseph, Ministry of Livestock and Fisheries Department, Vet Lab Kabete, P.O. Box 00625, Kangemi Nairobi 00000, Kenya, vetdept@todaysonline.com; hoyas@dvskabete.go.ke

MUSAI Lisa, 80 Abercromby Street, Port Spain P,O, Box 389, Trinidad y Tobago, aphmalmr@tstt.net.tt

MUSISI Frederick, Food & Agriculture Organization of the United Nationsn, 11 Naivasha Road, Sunninghill Johannesburg 2157, South Africa, fredlmusisi@yahoo.co.uk

NAEEM Khalid, National Reference Lab for Poultry Diseases, Animal Sciences Institute, NARC, Park Road, Islamabad 45500, Pakistan, naeem22@isb.comsats.net.pk

NASCIMIENTO Ricardo, Minidtry of Agriculture and Development Dep. Provincial dos Serviços de Veterinária Benguela, Po. Box. 571, Angola, ricardona16@yahoo.com.br

NEEDHAM Howard, European Centre For Disease Prevention and Control, Tomtebodavägan 11 A Solna, Stockholm, 171 83, Sweden, angus.nicoll@ecdc.eu.int

NEPOKLONOV Evgeny, CVO of the Russian Federation Orlikov Per. 1/11 Moscow, 107139, Russia, info@vet.mcx.ru

NETO Antonio, Ministry of Agriculture and Rural Development, Bairro Benfica, av. Diolinda Rodrigues, Laboratório Regional de Veterinária Huila Lubango, PO Box. 405, Italy, tony_r_neto@yahoo.com.br

NG Lip Tet, Agriculture, Fisheries and Conservation Department, Room 708, 7/F, Cheung Sha Wan Government Offices, 303 Road Kowloon, Hong Kong SAR, China, liptet_ng@afcd.gov.hk

NICOLI Pier Andra, Az. ULSS 18 di Rovigo Viale Tre Martiri n. 89, Rovigo 45100, Italy, veter.ro@azisanrovigo.it

NISI Raffaella, Istituto Zooprofilattico Sperimentale delle Venezie, Viale dell'Università 10 Legnaro, Padua 35020, Italy, mmandelli@izsvenezie.it

NORTHOFF Erwin, FAO, Viale delle Terme di Caracalla, Roma 00153, Italy, erwin.northoff@fao.org

ODENDAAL Mike, Rainbow Chickens, PO Box 1965, Rustenburg, Northwest Province 0300, South Africa, mikeo@rcf.co.za

OLIVIER Adriaan, SA Ostrich Business Chamber, PO Box 952, Oudtshoorn 6620, South Africa, admin@saobc.co.za

OLSEVSKIS Edvins, Food and Veterinary Service, Peldu 30, Riga, LV-1010, Latvia, edvins.olsevskis@pvd.gov.lv

ONITA Iuliana, Institute for Diagnosis and Animal Health, Dr. Staicovici street, 63 Bucharest, sector 5, Bucharest 050557, Romania, onita.iuliana@idah.ro

ORDONEZ German, CESAC Carretera Castellvell, s/n REUS, 43206, Spain, gordonez@cesac.org

ORTALI Giovanni, Veronesi Corte Pellegrina, San Martino Buon Albergo, Verona 37036, Italy, giovanni.ortali@veronesi.it

OSINGA Klass Johan, International Organisation of Agricultural Producers (IFAP), PO Box 186, Drachten 9200, Netherlands, kjosinga@ltonoord.nl

OZDARENDELI Aykut, Firat University Veterinary Medicine Department of Virology, Elazig 23119, Turkey, aozdarendeli@firat.edu.tr

PITTMAN Maria, European Commission, Rue Froissart 101, office 3/84, Brussels 1049, Belgium, maria.pittman@ec.europa.eu

PANT Ganesh Raj, Central Veterinary Laboratory, Tripureshwor Kathmandu 00977, Nepal, ganeshrajpant@yahoo.co.uk

PASSARINI Gastone, ASL 20 Verona, Via S. d'Acquisto 7, Verone, 37121 Italy, gastone.passarini@ulss20.verona.it

PATIL Mangesh, Venkateshwara Hatcheries Private Limited, 1206/18/B, Dealing Corner, 2nd Floor, Jangali Maharaj Road, Opposite Sambhaji Park Pune, Maharashtra 411 005, India, dr_mangesh@hotmail.com

PATTA Gian Paolo, Ministero della Salute, Lungotevere Ripa 1, Roma 00153, Italy, g.patta@sanita.it

PEDGAONKAR Prassana, Venkateshwara Hatcheries Private Limited, 1206/18/B, Dealing Corner, 2nd Floor, Jangali Maharaj Road, Opp. Sambhaji Park, Pune, Maharashtra 400 005, India, pgpedgaonkar@hotmail.com

PEDICONE Rossella, ConAv - Consorzio Zoo Avicunicolo soc. coop., Via Battuti Rossi 6/a, Forlì 47100, Italy, r.pedicone@avitalia.it

PERDUE Michel, WHO, 20 Appia Way, Geneva 1211, Switzerland, perduem@who.int

PEREDA Ariel, Instituto Nacional de Tecnología Agropecuaria (INTA) CC77, Castelar Pcia, Buenos Aires 1712, Argentina, apereda@cnia.inta.gov.ar

PERELMAN Beny, Abic Veterinary Products, Abic-Teva Industrial Area, West Beit Shemesh, Israel 9910, benny.perlman@teva.co.il

PERK Shimon, Kimron Veterinary Institute, Bet Dagan, PO Box 12, Israel 50250, shimonpr@moag.gov.il

PETITOT Henri, Afssa, 13, rue des Turlures, 77920 Samois-sur-Seine, France, henri.petitot@parimutuel.fr

PEYRE Marisa, CIRAD, Campus International de Baillarguet, TA A16/E, Montpellier 34398 Cedex 5, France, marisa.peyre@cirad.fr

PERLER Lukas, Swiss Federal Veterinary Office, Schwarzenburgstrasse 155, Bern CH-3003, Switzerland, lukas.perler@bvet.admin.ch

PETROVIC Nead, Veterinary Directorate, Ministry of Agriculture, Forestry and Water Management, Omladinskih brigada 1, Belgrade 11000, Serbia, nenadvet@gmail.com

PEYRE Marisa, CIRAD, Campus International de Baillarguet, TA A16/E Montpellier 34398 Cedex 5, France, marisa.peyre@cirad.fr

PFEFFER Caroline, Merial, 29 avenue Tony Garnier, Lyon, 69007, France, caroline.pfeffer@merial.com

PIAZZA Valentina, European Commission, Rue Belliard 232-9/06, Bruxelles 1040, Belgium, valentina.piazza@ec.europa.eu

PICCIRILLO Alessandra, Veterinary Medicine Faculty, University of Padua, Viale dell' Università 16, Legnaro (PD), 35020, Italy, alessandra.piccirillo@unipd.it

PICKETT Heather, Compassion in World, Farming River Court, Mill Lane Godalming, Surrey, GU7 1EZ, United Kingdom, heather@ciwf.co.uk

PIENNAR Ana, Department of Agriculture, Directorate Animal Health, P/Bag X138 Pretoria 0001, South Africa, carineP@nda.agric.za

PINTER Fabio, AULSS N. 22 Regione Veneto, via Ospedale n. 5, Villafranca di Verona 37069, Italy, fpinter@ulss22.ven.it

PINTO Julio, FAO, Viale delle Terme di Caracalla, Rome 00153, Italy, julio.pinto@fao.org

PIRAK Michael, Ministry of Agriculture, Afula Regional Poultry Lab., Hagilboa St. 30 Afula, 18100, Israel, mpirak@walla.co.il

PITTMAN Maria, European Commission, Health and Consumer Protection Directorate-General, Rue Froissart 101, B-1049 Brussels, maria.pittman@ec.europa.eu

PIZZUTO Matteo Samuele, Istituto Zooprofilattico Sperimentale delle Venezie, Viale dell'Università 10 Legnaro, Padua 35020, Italy, mpizzuto@izsvenezie.it

POLMAN Paula, Dutch Smallholders Association, Erichemsekade 11, Buren 4116 GD, Netherlands, paula.polman@planet.nl

PORCARI Marco, Via Malvicino 44 29015 Castel Giovanni - Piacenza, Italy,

POST Lyndel, The Australian Government, Department of Agriculture, Fisheries and Forestry, DAFF, GPO Box 858, Canberra, 2601, Australia, lyndel.post@daff.gov.au

POURQUIER Philiphe, ID VET, 167 Rue Medhi BenBarka, Zone Garosud, Montpellier 34070, France, philippe.pourquier@id-vet.com

POZZATO Nicola, IZSVE Via S.Giacomo, 5 Verona 37135, Italy, npozzato@izsvenezie.it

PRAJITNO Teguh, JAPFA COMFEED Wisma Millenia 5th Floor, Jalan M.T. Haryono Kav 16 Jakarta, 12810, Indonesia, teguhyp@japfacomfeed.co.id

PRANDINI Francesco, Merial Animal Health, Milanofiori, Strada 6, Palazzo E/5, Assago (MI) 20090, Italy, francesco.prandini@merial.com

PUGGIONI Giantonella, Istituto Zooprofilattico Sperimentale della Sardegna, via Duca degli Abruzzi n. 8, Sassari 07100, Italy, giantonella.puggioni@izs-sardegna.it

PULICI Laura, IZSVe Viale dell'Università, 10 Legnaro 35020, Italy, lpulici@izsvenezie.it

PURWANTO Bundi, PT Medion Jl. Babakan Ciparay No 282 Bandung, 40223, Indonesia, budi_p@medion.co.id

RAO Srinivas, VRC/NIAID/NIH, 40 Convent Drive, Room 1407, Bethesda, MD, 20892, USA, srao1@mail.nih.gov

RATANANAKORN Laddawalaya, Department of Livestock Development, 69/1 Phayathai Road, Bangkok 10400, Thailand, laddawalaya_r@dld.go.th; ladrat12@hotmail.com

REFAAT Mahmoud, IFT, Mokattam, Cairo, 11439, Egypt, technical@ift-online.com

RETNO Felicitas, PT Medion, Jl Raya Batujarjar no 29 Bandung, 40552, Indonesia, diyanti_r@medion.co.id

RIBO Oriol, EFSA Largo natale Palli 5/A, Parma 43100, Italy, oriol.ribo@efsa.europa.eu

RODRIGUEZ Fabiola, Instituto Colombiano Agropecuario ICA, Avenida 39#14-57 apartamento 302, Bogota 01, Colombia, fabiola.rodriguez@ica.gov.co

ROEDER Peter, FAO, Rome Lazio, 00100, Italy, peter4.roeder@fao.org

ROJO Francisco, Merial, Av. de las Fuentes No. 66, Parque Industrial FINSA, El Marques, Queretaro 76246, Mexico, Francisco.Rojo@Merial.com

ROMERO Bernardo, Merial Av. de las Fuentes No. 66, Parque Industrial FINSA, El Marques, Queretaro 76246, Mexico, Bernardo.Romero@Merial.com

ROMLAMDUAN Narin, Bangkok Agro -Industrial Product plc (CPF), 29/2 Moo 9 Suwintawong Rd, Nongjok, Bangkok 10530, Thailand, narin@cpf.co.th, narin49@gmail.com

RONG Wei, Animal Health Standard and Regulation Department, China, weirong@epizoo.org

ROSSI Alessandro, Stationsstrasse 12 CH-3097 Liebefeld- Bern, Switzerland, alessandro-rossi@idexx.com

ROTH James, Institute for International Cooperation in Animal Biologics, College of Veterinary Medicine, Iowa State University, Ames, Iowa, 50011, USA, jaroth@iastate.edu

ROTTA Giuliana, AIA-VERONESI San Martino, Buon Albergo - Verona 37036, Italy, giuliana.rotta@aia-spa.it

ROUMIANTZEFF Micha, 1, rue Dangon, 69004 Lyon, France, micharou@numericable.fr

ROYALS Michael, Europlex building, VI floor, ul.Pulawska 17 02, 515 Warsaw, Poland, royals@pharmajet.com

RUDOLF Miriam, Friedrich-Loeffler-Institut, Federal Research Institute for Animal Health, Reference Laboratory for Avian Influenza, Boddenblick 5a Greifswald, Insel Riems, 17439, Germany, miriam.rudolf@fli.bund.de

RUGBJERG Helene, Danish Veterinary and Food Administration, Moerkhoej Bygade 19, Soeborg, 2860, Denmark, hru@fvst.dk

RUSSELL Leon, World Veterinary Association, 33 Linda Lane, College Station, Texas 77845, USA, lrussell@cvm.tamu.edu

RUTILI Domenico, Istituto Zooprofilattico Sperimentale Dell'Umbria e delle Marche, Via G. Salvemini 1, Perugia 06126, Italy, d.rutili@izsum.it, s.fiorucci@izsum.it

SAFRONOVA Alexandra, CVO of the Russian Federation, Orlikov Per. 1/11, Moscow,107139, Russia, info@vet.mcx.ru

SAINT PIERRE Christophe, SEPPIC, Tour Kupka, C 7 Boulevard Frank Kupka, Paris La Defense Cedex 92039, France, christophe.saintpierre@airliquide.com

SALAH ELDIN Hatem, IFT St. no. 9, Block 6103, Mokattam, Cairo 11439, Egypt, technical@ift-online.com

SALVELLI Alessandro, A.S.L.22 Bussolengo (Vr), Via Roma 2, Castelnuovo del Garda 37014, Italy, sandrosalvelli@hotmail.com

SAMINA Itzchak, Kimron Veterinary Institute, PO Box 12, Beit-Dagan 50250, Israel, isami@moag.gov.il

SAMOREK Elzbieta, National Veterinary Resaearch Institute, AL. Partyzantow 57, Pulawy 24-100, Poland, elsam@piwet.pulawy.pl

SANDERS Richard, The Organic Research Centre, Elm Farm, Hamstead Marshall Newbury RG20 0HR, United Kingdom, richard.s@efrc.com

SANTUCCI Vincenzo Ugo, Ministry oh Health, Piazza Marconi 25, Rome 00144, Italy, u.santucci@sanita.it

SARTOR Alassandra, Istituto Zooprofilattico Sperimentale delle Venezie, Viale dell'Università 10 Legnaro, Padua 35020, Italy, asartor@izsvenezie.it

SAVIC Vladimir, Croatian Veterinary Institute, Poultry Centre, Heinzelova 55, Zagreb 10000, Croatia, vsavichr@yahoo.com

SAWITRI Elly, Directorate General of Livestock Services, Ministry of Agriculture Jalan Harsono Room No. 3 Ragunan, Jakarta 12550, Indonesia, elly@deptan.go.id

SCHOELL Kerstin, GTZ GmbH Dag-Haemmerskjoeld,Weg 1-5, Eschborn, 65760, Germany, kerstin.schoell@gtz.de

SCHOUSTRA Willem, FAO, Rome Viale delle Terme di Caracalla, Rome 00153, Italy, willem.schoustra@fao.org

SCHWABENBAUER Karin, FAO Rome Viale delle Terme di Caracalla Rome 00153, Italy, karin.schwabenbauer@fao.org

SCOLAMACCHIA Francesca, Istituto Superiore di Sanità, Viale Regina Elena 299, Rome 00161, Italy, francesca.scolamacchia@iss.it

SECK Boubacar M., FAO, BP 1317, Bamako 99999, Mali, bmseck@gmail.com

SENNE Dennis, USDA, APHIS, VS, NVSL 1800 Dayton Avenue P O Box 844, Ames, IA 50010, USA, Dennis.A.Senne@aphis.usda.gov

SERIC Sabina, Veterinary faculty Sarajevo, Zmaja od Bosne 90, Sarajevo 71 000, Bosnia & Herzegobina, sabina_seric@hotmail.com

SERRATOSA Jordi, EFSA, Largo natale Palli 5/A, Parma 43100, Italy, jordi.serratosa@efsa.europa.eu

SESTI Luiz, CEVA Saúde Animal, Rua Santa Justina 660, Vila Olímpia, São Paulo / SP, 04545-042, Brazil, luiz.sesti@cevabrasil.com.br

SHALABY Mohamed, Faculty of Veterinary Medicine,Cairo University Giza Sequare Egypt, Giza, 12211, Egypt, mshalaby@link.net

SHAW John, USDA/APHIS, 4700 River Road, Unit 33, Riverdale, Maryland, 20737, USA, john.l.shaw@aphis.usda.gov

SHTJEFNI Valentin, Institute of Food Safety and Veterinary Research, Aleksander Moisiu No. 82, Tirana, Albania, valentinshtjefni@yahoo.com

SIHVONEN Liisa, Evira, Virology Research Unit Mustialankatu 3, Helsinki FI-00790, Finland, liisa.sihvonen@evira.fi

SILVANO Maistro, ULSS n.4, Alto Vicentino, via Rasa n.9, 36016 Thiene, Italy, smaistro@ulss4.veneto.it

SIMS Les, Asia Pacific Veterinary Information Services Pty Ltd PO Box344 Palm Cove Qld, Australia 4879, apvis@bigpond.net.au

SINCLAIR Marna, Dept of Agriculture, Western Cape Province, South Africa, Private Bag X1, Elsenburg 7607, South Africa, MARNAS@ELSENBURG.COM

SLAVEC Brigita, Institute for Poultry Diseases, Veterinary Faculty Ljubljana, Cesta v Mestni Log 47, Ljubljana SI 1000, Slovenia, brigita.slavec@vf.uni-lj.si

SLINGENBERGH Jan, FAO, Viale delle Terme di Caracalla Roma, 00153, Italy, jan.slingenbergh@fao.org

SMIETANKA Krysztof, National Veterinary Research Institute, al. Partyzantow 57, Pulawy 24-100, Poland, ksmiet@piwet.pulawy.pl

SOARES Roberto, Ceva Sante Animale, 159 av. G. Pompidou, BP126, Libourne 33501, France, roberto.soares@ceva.com

SODIKIN Erizal, Embassy of the Republic of Indonesia, Via Campania 55, Rome 00187, Italy, erizalsodikin79@yahoo.com

SOTGIA Stefano, ECGrange, FVO 1/124, Dunsany County, Meath, Ireland, stefano.sotgia@ec.europa.eu

SOUMAH Soriba, Ministère de la Santé Publique, Boulevard du Commerce, Conarky 6003, République de Guinee, popuenviron20052010@yahoo.fr

SPERATI Luigi, Veronesi Corte Pellegrina, San Martino Buon Albergo, Verona 37036, Italy, luigi.sperati@aia-spa.it

STANOJEVIC Slobodan, Veterinary Directorate, Ministry of Agriculture, Forestry and Water Management, Omladinskih brigada 1, Belgrade 11000, Serbia, slavavet@yahoo.com

STARK Katharina, Royal Veterinary College, Dept.Vet.Clin.Sci., Hawkshead Lane, North Mymms Hertfordshive, AL 97TA, United Kingdom, kstaerk@rvc.ac.uk

STEENSELS Mieke, Veterinary and Agrochemcial Research Center (VAR), Groeselenberg 99, Brussels 1180, Belgium, miste@var.fgov.be

STEGEMAN Arjan, Utrecht University, Yalelaan 7, Utrecht 3584 CL, Netherlands, j.a.stegeman@vet.uu.nl

STEINMETZ Philippe, European Commission, Rue Froissart 101, Office 3/84, Brussels 1049, Belgium, philippe.steinmetz@ec.europa.eu

STYLES Darrel, USDA APHIS, 4700 River Road, Unitl 84,Riverdale, MD 20737, USA, darrel.k.styles@aphis.usda.gov

SUAREZ David, Southeast Poultry Research Laboratory, USDA, 934 College Station Rd, Athens, GA 30605, Italy, dsuarez@seprl.usda.gov

SUDIRMAN Doctor, Sierad Produces, Plaza City View, Building Jalan Keman Timur No. 22, Jakarta Selatan, Indonesia, teguyp@japfacomfeed.co.id

SUDSAKORN Pratuang, Animal Helath and Technical Service Office, CP Tower, 313 Silom Road, Bangkok 10500, Thailand, pratuang@cpf.go.th

SULTAN Hishman, IFT St. no. 9, Block 6103, Mokattam Cairo, 11439, Egypt, technical@ift-online.com

SWAYNE David E., US Department of Agriculture 934 College Station Rd Athens, Georgia 30605, USA, dswayne@seprl.usda.gov

TAHA Mohamed, Egyptian Serum & Vaccine Institute Mokattam, Cairo, 11439, Egypt, technical@ift-online.com

TANAKA Robert, US Department of Agriculture USDA-APHIS, American Embassy, Boltzmanngasse 16, Vienna, A-1090, Austria, Robert.T.Tanaka@aphis.usda.gov

TARRÉS-CALL Jordi, Fort Dodge Veterinaria SA, Ctra. de Camprodon s/n, Vall de Bianya (Girona) 17813, Spain, tarresj@fdah.com

TAVARES Patricia, Direcção Geral de Veterinária, Largo da Academia Nacional de Belas Artes, nº 2 Lisboa 1249-105, Portugal, psantos@dgv.min-agricultura.pt

TERREGINO Calogero, Istituto Zooprofilattico delle Venezie, Viale dell'Università 10, Legnaro (Padua) 35020, Italy, cterregino@izsvenezie.it

TERRELL Alan, USDA-APHIS-International Services, AM Embassy, Unit 3500, APO AA 34030, USA, alan.terrell@aphis.usda.gov

TERRERA Maria Victoria, SENASA- Dilab,,Av.Fleming 1653, Buenos Aires, 1640, Argentina, mterrera@senasa.gov.ar

TERVELL Margareta, Swedish Board of Agriculture, Jordbruksverket Vallgatan 8, Joenkoeping, S-551 82, Sweden, margareta.tervell@sjv.se

THERON Louis, Sangiro PO Box 74, Broederstroom, 0240, South Africa, louis@sangiro.co.za

TO Lan Thanh, National Center for Veterinary Diagnosis 11, Lane 78, Giai Phong Street, Vietnam, thanhto@fpt.vn; tznt2002@yahoo.com

TOLLERSRUD Tore, National Veterinary Institute, PO Box 8156 Dep, Oslo, 0033, Norway, tore.tollersrud@vetinst.no

TOSCANI Tonino, AMADORI, Via Bonfadina 9, Cazzago S. Martino, 25046, Italy, tonino.toscani@amadori.it

TRIPODI Astrid, FAO, Viale delle Terme di Caracalla Roma, 00153, Italy, astrid.tripodi@fao.org

TROSTLE Murray, US Agency for International Development, 6336 Demme Place, Springfield/Virginia, 22150, USA, mtrostle@usaid.gov

TUMINO Giovanni, Istituto Zooprofilattico sperimentale della Sicilia, C/da Nunziata, Ragusa 97100, Italy, giovanni.tumino@izssicilia.it

TURLÀ Roberto, A.S.L.n. 7,Ragusa, via Risorgimento n. 92, Modica 97015, Italy, r.turla@ausl7.rg.it

USBERTI Rodingo, Con. Av. Piazzale Foro Piazzale Foro Boario, Forlì 47100, Italy, rodingovet@libero.it

VALLAT Bernard, OIE, 12 rue de Prony, 75017 Paris, France, oie@oie.int

VAN AARLE Paul, Intervet International bv, Wim de Körverstraat 35, P.O Box 31, Boxmeer 5830 AA, Netherlands, paul.vanaarle@intervet.com

VAN DE LAAR Armand, Organisation for Economic Co-operation and Development, 2 rue André-Pascal, Paris 75775 Cedex 16, France, armand.vandelaar@oecd.org

VAN LANGEN Herman, Food and Consumer Product Safety Authority, PO Box 19506, Den Haag, 2500 CM, Netherlands, herman.van.langen@vwa.nl

VAYUCHOTE Nopporn, Betagro Group 59/111-112 Thung Song Hong, Laksi, Bangkok 10210, Thailand, nopporn@betagro.com

VEITS Jutta, Friedrich Loeffler Institut, Boddenblick 5a, Greifswald-Insel, Riems 17493, Germany, jutta.veits@fli.bund.de

VERONESI Giordano, AIA Agricola Italiana Alimentare, Via San Antonio n° 60, San Martino Buon Albergo, Verona 37036, Italy, aia@aia-spa.it

VERONESI Bruno, AIA Agricola Italiana Alimentare,Via San Antonio n° 60, San Martino Buon Albergo, Verona 37036, Italy, aia@aia-spa.it

VERONESI Carlo, AIA Agricola Italiana Alimentare,Via San Antonio n° 60, San Martino Buon Albergo, Verona 37036, Italy, aia@aia-spa.it

VERZHYKHOVSKIY Oleksandr, State Department of Veterinary Medicine, Ministry of Agricultural Policy of Ukraine 24, Khreschatik str. Kiev 01001, Ukraine, verzh@minapk.gov.ua

VICENZONI Gaddo, Istituto Zooprofilattico Sperimentale delle Venezie, Viale dell'Università 10 Legnaro, Padua 35020, Italy, gaddovic@izsvenezie.it

VICTORIA Gustavo, Investigación Aplicada, S.A. de C.V. 7 Norte 416 Tehuacán, Puebla, 75700, Mexico, gvictoria@grupoidisa.com

VILLAREAL Cesar, (SENASICA, SAGARPA), Mexico, Municipio Libre 377, 6A, col.Sta. Cruz Atoyac Ciudad de México 03310, Mexico, coor.tec@senasica.sagarpa.gob.mx; clvillarrealch02@yahoo.com.mx

VITASEK Josef, State Veterinary Administration, Slezska 7, Praha 2 Prague, 120 00, Czech Republic, j.vitasek@svscr.cz

VLADIMIR Zelnik, Lohmann Animal Health GmbH & Co., KG Heinz-Lohmann-Strasse 4, Cuxhaven 27472, Germany, vladimir.zelnik@lah.de

VON TROTT ZU SOLZ Wilhelm, Boehringer Ingelheim Vetmedica, Calle 30 No. 2614 Zona Industrial, Guadalajara, Jalisco, 44940, Mexico, TROTT@ing.boehringer-ingelheim.com

VOSS Matthias, Lohmann Tierzucht GmbH, Am Seedeich 9-11, Cuxhaven, D-27472, Germany, voss@ltz.de

VOSTINAKOVA Veronika, State Veterinary Institute Prague, Sidlistni 24 Praha 6, Lysolaje, Prague 165 03, Czech Republic, vosver@centrum.cz

WACHARONKE Chai, Knack Kohland CO. Ltd, 1550 Thanapoom Tower, 16th Floor, New Petchaburi RD, Makasan Ratchatevee, Bangkok 10400, Thailand, chai@kohlan.com

WEAVER John, FAO, 7th Floor, Menara Thamrin, Jl Thamrin, Jakarta 10250, Indonesia, john.weaver@fao.org

WEIJTENS Martijn, Ministry of Agruculture, Nature and Food Quality Bezuidenhoutseweg 73 Den Haag, 2500 EK, Netherlands, m.j.b.m.weijtens@minlnv.nl

WEINANDY Herbert, Federal Ministry of Food, Agriculture and Consumer Protection, Rochusstrasse 1, Bonn 53123, Germany, Herbert.Weinandy@bmelv.bund.de

WIJASZKA Tadeusz, National Veterinary Research Institute Al. Partyzantow 57, Pulawy 24 -100, Poland, T.Wijaszka@hotmail.com

WOOLDRIDGE Marion, Centre for Epidemiology & Risk Analysis, VLA (Weybridge), Addlestone, Surrey KT15 3NB, United Kingdom, m.wooldridge@vla.defra.gsi.gov.uk

YASSER Mohamed, IFT St. no. 9, Block 6103, Mokattam Cairo 11439, Egypt, technical@ift-online.com

ZAMPAGLIONE Maria, OIE, 12 rue de Prony, 75017 Paris, France, m.zampaglione@oie.int

ZEPEDA Christobal, CEAH-OIE Collaborating Center for Disease Surveillance and Risk Analysis, 2150 Centre Ave. Bldg. B, Fort Collins, Colorado, 80526, USA, cristobal.zepeda@aphis.usda.gov

ZHIZHONG Zhizhong, Shandong Agricultural University, #61 Daizong street, Taian, Shandong 271018, China, zzcui@sdau.edu.cn

ZRELLI Malek, Ministère de l'Agriculture, 30 rue Alain Savary, Tunis, 1002, Tunisia, zrelli.malek@iresa.agrinet.tn

Index of Authors

Developments in Biological Standardization

Vol. 36	Washington DC, 1976	Freeze-Drying of Biological Products
Vol. 37	Geneva, 1976	Standardization of Cell Substrates for the Production of Virus Vaccines
Vol. 38	London, 1977	Biological Preparations in the Treatment of Cancer
Vol. 39	Geneva, 1977	Influenza Immunization
Vol. 40	Marburg, 1977	Standardization of Rabies Vaccines for Human Use Produced in Tissue Culture (Rabies III)
Vol. 41	Guadeloupe, 1978	Vaccines in the Developing Countries
Vol. 42	Paris, 1978	Second General Meeting of ESACT
Vol. 43	Brussels, 1978	Immunization: Benefit Versus Risk Factors
Vol. 44	Villars, 1979	Test methods for the Quality Control of Plasma Proteins
Vol. 45	San Antonio, 1979	The Standardization of Animals to Improve Biomedical Research, Production and Control
Vol. 46	Oxford, 1979	Third General Meeting of ESACT
Vol. 47	Bilthoven, 1980	Reassessment of Inactivated Poliomyelitis Vaccine
Vol. 48	Geneva, 1980	Standardization of Albumin, Plasma Substitutes and Plasmapheresis
Vol. 49	Leetown, 1981	Fish Biologics: Serodiagnostics and Vaccines
Vol. 50	Heidelberg, 1981	The Use of Heteroploid and Other Cell Substrates for the Production of Biologicals
Vol. 51	Lyons, 1981	Immunization of Adult Birds with Inactivated Oil Adjuvant Vaccines
Vol. 52	Lyons, 1981	Herpes Virus of Man and Animal: Standardization of Immunological Procedures
Vol. 53	Dublin, 1982	Enteric Infections in Man and Animals: Standardization of Immunological Procedures
Vol. 54	Athens, 1982	Viral Hepatitis: Standardization in Immunoprophylaxis of Infections by Hepatitis Viruses
Vol. 55	Copenhagen, 1982	Fifth General Meeting of ESCAT
Vol. 56	Algiers, 1983	Third International Symposium on Brucellosis
Vol. 57	Paris, 1983	Monoclonal Antibodies: Standardization of their Characterization and Use
Vol. 58	Budapest, 1983	International Symposium on BCG Vaccines and Tuberculins
Vol. 59	Geneva, 1983	Standardization and Control of Biologicals Produced by Recombinant DNA Technology
Vol. 60	Gardone Riviera, 1984	Production and Exploitation of Existing and New Animal Cell Substrates
Vol. 61	Geneva, 1984	Proceedings of the Fourth International Symposium on Pertussis
Vol. 62	Stockholm, 1985	Diagnostics and Vaccines for Parasitic Diseases
Vol. 63	San Francisco, 1985	Use and Standardization of Chemically Defined Antigens
Vol. 64	London, 1985	Reduction of Animal Usage in the Development and Control of Biological Products
Vol. 65	Amsterdam, 1985	Use and Standardization of Combined Vaccines

Vol. 66	Vienna, 1985	Advances in Animal Cell Technology: Cell Engineering, Evaluation and Exploitation
Vol. 67	Melbourne, 1986	Standardization in Blood Fractionation Including Coagulation Factors
Vol. 68	Geneva, 1986	Cells - Products - Safety
Vol. 69	London, 1987	Cytokines Laboratory and Clinical Evaluation
Vol. 70	Arlington, VA, 1988	Continuous Cell Lines as Substrates for Biologicals
Vol. 71	Utrecht, 1989	Monoclonal Antibodies for Therapy, Prevention and In vivo Diagnosis of Human Disease
Vol. 72	Annecy, 1989	Progress in Animal Retroviruses
Vol. 73	Shizuoka, 1990	Pertussis: Evaluation and Research on Acellular Pertussis Vaccines
Vol. 74	Bethesda, MD, 1990	Biological Product Freeze-Drying and Formulation
Vol. 75	London, 1990	Virological Aspects of the Safety of Biological Products
Vol. 76	Bethesda, MD, 1991	Continuous Cell Lines - An International Workshop on Current Issues
Vol. 77	Annecy, 1991	Standardization of the Immunopharmacology of Natural and Synthetic Immunomodulators
Vol. 78	Bethesda, MD, 1991	Poliovirus Attenuation: Molecular Mechanisms and Practical Aspects
Vol. 79	Ploufragan, 1992	The First Steps Towards an International Harmonization of Veterinary Biologicals: 1993 and Free Circulation of Vaccines within the EEC
Vol. 80	Heidelberg, 1992	Transmissible Spongiform Encephalopathies - Impact on Animal and Human Health
Vol. 81	Cannes, 1992	Virological Safety Aspects of Plasma Derivatives
Vol. 82	Albany NY, 1993	Recombinant Vectors in Vaccine Development
Vol. 83	Annecy, 1993	Genetic Stability and Recombinant Product Consistency
Vol. 84	Langen, 1993	Non-Target Effects of Live Vaccines
Vol. 85	Santa Fé, NM, 1994	Genetics of Streptococci, Enterococci and Lactococci
Vol. 86	Langen, 1994	Replacement, Reduction and Refinement of Animal Experiments in the Development and Control of Biological Products
Vol. 87	Geneva, 1995	New Approaches to Stabilisation of Vaccines Potency
Vol. 88	Bethesda, MD, 1995	Viral Safety and Evaluation of Viral Clearance from Biopharmaceutical Products
Vol. 89	Rome, 1995	Pertussis Vaccine Trials
Vol. 90	Oslo, 1996	Fish Vaccinology
Vol. 91	San Francisco, CA, 1996	Development of Specifications for Biotechnology Pharmaceuticals Products
Vol. 92	Bergen, 1996	Modulation of the Immune Response to Vaccine Antigens
Vol. 93	Annecy, 1996	Safety of Biological Products Prepared from Mammalian Cell Culture
Vol. 94	Bethesda, MD, 1997	Simian Virus 40 (SV40): A Possible Human Polyomavirus
Vol. 95	Paris, 1997	Preclinical and Clinical Development of New Vaccines
Vol. 96	Washington, DC, 1995	Characterization of Biotechnology Pharmaceutical Products
Vol. 97	London, 1997	Biological Characterization and Assay of Cytokines and Growth Factors
Vol. 98	London, 1997	Inactivated Influenza Vaccines Prepared in Cell Culture
Vol. 99	Strasbourg, 1998	Animal Sera, Animal Sera Derivatives and Substitutes Used in the Manufacture of Pharmaceuticals: Viral Safety and Regulatory Aspects
Vol. 100	Geneva, 1998	A Celebration of 50 Years of Progress in Biological Standardization and Control at WHO
Vol. 101	London, 1998	Alternatives to Animals in the Development and Control of Biological Products for Human and Veterinary Use

Developments in Biologicals

Vol. 102	San Francisco, CA, 1999	Advances in Transfusion Safety
Vol. 103	Annecy, 1999	Physico-Chemical Procedures for the Characterization of Vaccines
Vol. 104	Langen, 1999	Development and Clinical Progress of DNA Vaccines
Vol. 105	Paris, 2000	Progress in Polio Eradication: Vaccine Strategies for the End Game
Vol. 106	Rockville, MD, 2000	Evolving Scientific and Regulatory Perspectives on Cell Substrates for Vaccine Development
Vol. 107	London, 2000	The Design and Analysis of Potency Assays for Biotechnology Products
Vol. 108	Langen, 2001	Advances in Transfusion Safety
Vol. 109	Washington, DC, 2000	Biologics 2000 – Comparability of Biotechnology Products
Vol. 110	Palm Cove, 2001	Orphan Vaccines – Bridging the Gap
Vol. 111	Utrecht, 2001	Advancing Science and Elimination of the Use of Laboratory Animals for Development and Control of Vaccines and Hormones
Vol. 112	Bethesda, MD, 2001	Immunogenicity of Therapeutic Biological Products
Vol. 113	Berlin, 2001	Process Validation for Manufacturing of Biologics and Biotechnology Products
Vol. 114	Ames, IA, 2002	Vaccines for OIE List A and Emerging Animal Diseases
Vol. 115	Bergen, 2002	Laboratory Correlates of Immunity to Influenza – A Reassessment,
Vol. 116	Los Angeles, CA, 2003	Development of Therapeutic Cancer Vaccines
Vol. 117	Langen, 2003	Consideration of Alternative Licensing Procedures for Vaccines for Minor Species, Minor Indications and Autogenous/Autologous Products
Vol. 118	Langen, 2003	PDA/EMEA European Virus Safety Forum
Vol. 119	Buenos Aires, 2004	Control of Infectious Animal Diseases by Vaccination
Vol. 120	Bethesda, MD, 2003	Advances in Transfusion Safety
Vol. 121	Bergen, 2003	Progress in Fish Vaccinology
Vol. 122	Bethesda, MD, 2003	State of the Art Analytical Methods for Characterization of Biological Products and Assessment of Comparability
Vol. 123	Rockville, MD, 2004	Vaccine Cell Substrates 2004
Vol. 124	Paris, France, 2005	OIE/FAO International Scientific Conference on Avian Influenza
Vol. 125	Kiev, Ukraine, 2005	First International Conference on Rabies in Europe
Vol. 126	Saint-Malo, France, 2005	New Diagnostic Technology: Applications in Animal Health and Biologics Controls
Vol. 127	Sydney, Australia, 2005	Advances in Transfusion Safety – Volume IV
Vol. 128	Florianopolis, Brazil, 2006	First International Conference of the OIE Reference Laboratories and Collaborating Centres
Vol. 129	Bergen, Norway, 2006	The OIE Global Conference on Aquatic Animal Health